Praise for The Tantru

"This is the toddler decoding manua. ...g ... As the mother of a three-year-old and a 20-month-old, I deal with a double dose of tantrums on a daily basis. This book has been a lifesaver in terms of how to understand the root causes and triggers of my kids' tantrums, how to process my own emotions during them, and how to handle (and even prevent) tantrums in the future. Dr. Hershberg somehow makes you feel listened to and validated simply through reading her words."
—*Sumana W., Los Angeles*

"Dr. Hershberg comes across like the smartest, most thoughtful of my 'mom friends'—and a funny one, too. She doesn't shy away from digging deep into the outsized emotions of little kids. I feel like a psychological supermom now, ready to handle anything my four- and two-year-olds throw my way!"
—*Ali M., Dobbs Ferry, New York*

"As a father of two, I found this to be an invaluable tool for living in the trenches with young kids. With warmth and humor, Dr. Hershberg assures you that you are not alone and describes strategies that work."
—*Chris D., Chatham, New Jersey*

"What a wonderful book! Dr. Hershberg writes with wisdom and humor about the experience of both child and parent as each of you struggles with the huge feelings unleashed in a tantrum. Her 'L words'—love and limits—are a timeless guide for those confusing moments when you feel torn about what to do next. Every parent of a toddler should read this book!"
—*Alicia F. Lieberman, PhD, author of*
The Emotional Life of the Toddler

"Witty and authentic—an invaluable resource for dealing with meltdowns, especially at inopportune times and places. Unlike most parenting books, this one is painfully realistic. Dr. Hershberg shares her own struggles to manage her toddlers' behavior, despite her considerable expertise as a child psychologist."
—*Joan L. Luby, MD, Director, Early Emotional*
Development Program, Washington University
School of Medicine in St. Louis

"Dr. Hershberg gives parents the ultimate gift of how to survive (and even prevent) tantrums. Her perspective as both a child psychologist and a mother is refreshing and easy to relate to. She takes you right into the eye of the storm to help you understand what is going on in your toddler's mind. A 'must read' for all moms and dads—keep this book in your parenting tool box."
—*Deena Blanchard, MD, MPH, pediatrician,*
New York City

THE TANTRUM SURVIVAL GUIDE

THE TANTRUM SURVIVAL GUIDE

Tune In to Your Toddler's Mind
(and Your Own) to Calm the Craziness
and Make Family Fun Again

Rebecca Schrag Hershberg, PhD

Foreword by Daniel J. Siegel, MD

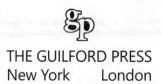

THE GUILFORD PRESS
New York   London

Library of Congress Cataloging-in-Publication Data

Names: Hershberg, Rebecca Schrag, author.
Title: The tantrum survival guide : tune in to your toddler's mind (and your
    own) to calm the craziness and make family fun again / Rebecca Schrag
    Hershberg ; foreword by Daniel J. Siegel.
Description: First Edition. | New York : The Guilford Press, 2019. | Includes
    bibliographical references and index.
Identifiers: LCCN 2018031473| ISBN 9781462537259 (hardback) | ISBN
    9781462529711 (paperback)
Subjects: LCSH: Temper tantrums in children. | Toddlers. | Child rearing. |
    BISAC: FAMILY & RELATIONSHIPS / Life Stages / Infants & Toddlers. |
    PSYCHOLOGY / Developmental / Child. | MEDICAL / Psychiatry / Child &
    Adolescent. | SOCIAL SCIENCE / Social Work.
Classification: LCC BF723.A4 H47 2018 | DDC 649/.123--dc23
LC record available at https://lccn.loc.gov/2018031473

For Henry and Zeke,
without whom there would be no book

And for Jon,
without whom there would be no Henry and Zeke

Contents

Foreword   ix

Acknowledgments   xi

Introduction   1

1 "You Haven't Seen a Tantrum Until You've Seen   13
My Toddler's Tantrums": When Should You Worry?

2 "Really? *This* Is What You're Going to Melt Down Over?":   23
Understanding Causes and Triggers

3 "What's Going On in That Curious Little Mind?":   43
Being Realistic about the Limitations of the Developing Brain

4 "Why Can't I Handle This?": Parental Expectations,   67
Baggage, and Emotions

5 "Maybe If Things Were Just a Bit Less Crazy on   91
the Home Front . . .": Family Dynamics and
the Foundation for Reducing Tantrums

6 "Of Course You'll Always Be My Sweet Little Baby   112
(Except Possibly When You Pee in the Bath on Purpose)":
Preserving the Authentic Connection with Your Toddler

7 "Who's Making the Rules Here?": Using Reasonable Structures 124
and Routines to Help Your Toddler Feel Secure

8 "OK. But. Now. What. Exactly. Should. I. *Do*?": Practical Strategies 139
for Preventing and Deescalating Tantrums

9 "Am I Making Things Worse?": Concrete Ways to Avoid 170
Knee-Jerk Responses and Other "Anti-Tools"
That Just Don't Work

10 "Please Just Go to Sleep, Already!": How to Reduce Tantrums 182
at Tough Times of Day, from Wake-Up to Bedtime

11 "How Many Times Can We Order Pizza for Dinner?" 198
(a.k.a. Another Aborted Trip to the Supermarket):
How to Reduce Tantrums in Tricky Settings, from the Big-Box
Store to the Playground and Beyond

12 "A Tantrum Is Quite Possibly the Last Thing I Need Right Now": 212
How to Reduce Tantrums under Difficult Circumstances,
from Travel to Moving to Divorce

Resources 231

Index 241

About the Author 250

Foreword

Imagine a guide that can offer you an accessible, scientifically sound foundation for understanding your young child's tantrums and then provide you accessible, practical, and effective ways to help connect with your child through the moments of meltdowns and tirades. This is the book you are about to dive into, written in clear, engaging, and well-timed humorous prose that will teach and reassure you all at once.

Raising children is one of the most challenging and important roles we will ever take on in life. The early years—especially the second to fifth years of life, the toddler and preschool period—are filled with developmental changes. These changes yield intense emotions and confusing behaviors that can challenge any parent to know what to do or how to make sense of the sudden shifts from calm to chaos. Sometimes it feels downright impossible to figure out how to respond in an effective way that will support the growth of a healthy child and maintain a strong and nurturing relationship with your child.

The wonderful creator of this smart book is not only a brilliant translator of the science of good relationships and the brain, but also an astute, humble, and hilarious observer of human nature. Rebecca Hershberg's experience as a practicing clinical psychologist provides her with illuminating stories from the trenches about real-life challenges of parenting young children. Her personal family life with two young ones at home also offers the immediacy of a parent's inner observations of the parenting journey—highlighting the research finding that the best first step of enhancing our connection with our children is to make sense of our own childhood experiences and how these have shaped our own development.

The first half of the book focuses on foundational concepts and science, the second leads you through practical steps and stories. Thus this important guide offers you a comprehensive way of not only surviving but thriving as a family in the face of the emotional turmoil we call tantrums—and shows how you can effectively navigate these challenging years with a sense of humility, humor, and mastery. Enjoy the journey ahead!

DANIEL J. SIEGEL, MD
Clinical Professor
UCLA School of Medicine

Acknowledgments

There are so many people to whom I owe a debt of gratitude for this book. First and foremost, I had always heard that editors can work magic, but Christine Benton and Kitty Moore exceeded my highest expectations, not only in their skills, but also—and perhaps even more so—with regard to their incredible kindness and support throughout the process. Also at The Guilford Press is Lucy Baker, who had the idea and made the connection in the first place: Thank you. Dr. Tara Peris, with her characteristic brilliant candor, supplied the quote around which the Introduction, and then so much of the book, was crafted. Thank you to Dr. Rahil Briggs, for taking a chance on me way back in the pre-KFC days, and to my colleagues at Healthy Steps at Montefiore (Dr. Miguelina Germán; Laura Krug, LCSW; Dr. Polina Umylny), for teaching me so much about working with the families of young children. Of course, going even further back in time, thank you to Dr. Alan Kazdin, for being my first mentor, one who has lived up to the title by supplying equal parts guidance, support, wisdom, and humor for over 20 years. I'm grateful to Dr. Elizabeth Cohen, for always pushing me to think big and be gentle on myself (simultaneously), and to Dr. Alison Locker, for bringing her vast knowledge, insight, and humor to Little House Calls. Brian Reisinger is responsible for the back cover photo, and The Dobbs Ferry Commune gets credit for keeping me sane on many a Sunday afternoon (and without sanity on Sunday, who can write on Monday?).

A new paragraph to emphasize my ongoing gratitude to the families with whom I've worked, and continue to work, for letting me into their most vulnerable parenting moments; it takes such courage to ask for help, and to remember, in our darkest, most frustrated moments, that we're all on this journey together.

A special thank-you—for everything—to my own parents: so loving, generous, and devoted, also complicated and imperfect. Descriptors that fit us all, although we only realize it when we become parents ourselves. Along those lines, never-ending gratitude to Henry and Zeke, for cracking my heart open in ways I never knew possible. Thank *you*, Henry, for your funny dancing, constant curiosity, and striking thoughtfulness. And thank *you*, Zeke, for your mushy hugs, sly looks, and daily reminders that you are my baby. I'm in awe every day that the two of you came from your daddy and me. And so lastly, to your daddy, Jon: Thank you for too many things to count. From day one, you told me I could do this. And so I could.

Introduction

Hi. I can't believe you pulled it off. You found a few minutes of downtime to start this book. I don't know whether you're reading after flopping onto the couch, or while standing at the kitchen counter clutching a cup of coffee or glass of wine, or once you've finally collapsed into bed (presuming you can keep your eyes open for even a few seconds). The fact that you're here, though, on this page with me, says a few things about where you're at in this moment. Most likely, within the last couple of hours— and undoubtedly within the past day or two—you have stood in front of a shrieking, stomping little human and felt like closing up shop and retreating. Although you're not accustomed to carrying around a white flag, you came close to taking the crumpled-up, snot-covered tissue out of your back pocket, waving it in the air, and surrendering to the three-foot-tall monster in your midst. And sure, there's a part of you that can laugh at that image, find humor in the fact that your kingdom has been taken hostage by a creature who somehow subsists solely on chicken nuggets and buttered noodles. Yet there are so many other emotions there as well: frustration, shame, powerlessness, anger, regret, guilt, rage, sadness, hopelessness. The feelings that arise in the wake of tantrums are no joke. Maybe you didn't, or don't, feel all of them, but even just one or two can pack a real punch and deserve to be acknowledged.

So perhaps it's this most recent showdown that led you—possibly in tears, or sweating, maybe with a hoarse voice, or a budding curiosity about how exactly one goes about giving one's kids up for adoption (kidding, mostly)—to this book. Or maybe it's just a general sense that things aren't working at home quite as well as they should or, at least, not the way you envisioned when you started out on this whole parenting adventure. You're an adoring parent—really and truly—and yet occasionally on your drive to work after a morning of mayhem you contemplate what it would feel like if you just kept driving . . . Or you're on the quiet car of the commuter train in the evening, realizing—not without some guilt—that it's become the part of your week that you treasure most. If only "Sorry, can't talk; I'm on the quiet car" was an excuse you could use more than twice a day. Or maybe your baby is growing up so fast that you want to get a bit of a head start— are the "terrible twos," the "threenage" years, and the "ferocious fours" really as tough as they say?

I get it. I do. I too am a parent. I have two little boys, Henry, almost four years old as I finish writing this book, and Zeke, who just turned two. They are 21 months apart. Did I mention I get it? I will never forget what happened over breakfast the very first morning I sat down to start writing this book in earnest. Henry was a bit over two and a half at the time. He decided there weren't enough raisins in his cinnamon raisin bagel, so my husband gave him a few more to spread on top of the cream cheese. Henry moved all of said raisins onto approximately one square inch of the bagel, then licked it bare before declaring he was done and had to go pee-pee. He promptly bolted out of the kitchen and up the stairs to find "Red Car," which, it seems, was absolutely essential for companionship prior to emp- tying his bladder. He couldn't find it (no surprise); it was in his crib, along with roughly 16 other toy cars (because who wouldn't want to sleep next to 17 small metal objects?). At that point, I raced up the stairs to find Red Car myself, so that Henry would make it to the toilet rather than peeing in his PJs. I left Zeke, then 11 months, in his high chair, at which point he realized—I soon discovered—that he could reach Henry's bagel with his cute little pudgy fingers and effectively rub cream cheese all over his ears and hair.

Because I'm an early childhood psychologist, however—one who was about to embark upon writing this book, no less!—I handled the entire epi- sode as a beacon of grace and serenity. When I finally found Red Car and handed it to Henry, I did so calmly, and with a smile (read: I thrust it into his palm with a "Here, OK? Here!" before sweeping him up and essentially throwing—ahem, placing—him onto the toilet). When I noticed Zeke had styled his hair with cream cheese, I giggled to myself, nuzzled his neck, gave him a quick bath, and snuggled him in a freshly washed towel before getting him dressed (read: I soaked the hair in question with a wet paper towel I'd used earlier to wipe the table, decided he was "clean enough," and stuffed him into the sweatpants he'd worn the day before and a slightly too small shirt, because whoever has the time it takes to switch the clothes in children's drawers as quickly as they grow?).

So yes, I am an early childhood psychologist, but no, that doesn't mean that I haven't been exactly where you are right now, with all that implies. I'd like to believe—and do—that my professional background, training, degree, and experience have gifted me with some helpful insights and tools for how to survive, and even enjoy, the toddler and preschool phases. I'm honored to have worked with numerous families—I say honored because it's an incredible privilege to have parents place their trust in me when it comes to the precious beings who own their hearts—and to have come up with an approach to thinking about young children and tantrums that is both accessible and helpful. Yet, because I'm also Mommy, I'm someone whose daily struggles and triumphs likely look a great deal like yours. Over the past year and a half, while devoting myself to writing this book, I was not only working in the field—seeing clients, giving talks, running workshops—but also living the work: pumping breast milk, surgically removing single bites from apples so as to salvage perfectly good fruit, and wrangling my kids into their clothes (Henry wants to pick out his own clothes, then he doesn't, then he does, then he decides walking with his pants around his ankles is riotously funny, then he falls and bumps his head, which of course typically happens right after I start changing Zeke's diaper, etc., etc.).

Is This Book for You?

If you're a parent who's struggling with your child's tantrums, the answer is yes. But let me get a little more specific about what I mean by "parent" and "child."

- *Parent*: I use this word throughout the book to describe anyone who is caring for a child, be that a biological parent, an adoptive or foster parent, a grandmother, an uncle, or a babysitter. "Parent" is simply shorthand for any one, or all, of these caregivers.

- *Child*: Tantrums typically begin around 18 months of age and last (although generally waning in frequency, duration, and severity) until age four or five years. This does not mean that older children, teenagers, and even adults never have tantrums. But the kinds of episodes we're discussing are most common between the ages of two and four, and so the children I focus on in the book generally fall within this range. That said, I'm confident that the understanding you gain from the following pages will serve you well for years to come, because it will give you a foundation in the emotional development of children and provide insight into their internal lives well beyond the arena of tantrums.

It's often asserted, as a rationale for addressing behavioral and emotional issues in early childhood rather than putting it off, that little kids have little problems and big kids have big problems. The thing that sometimes gets overlooked, however, is that the substance of these problems and the family dynamics underlying them frequently remain somewhat the same as the child grows. For example, both three-year-olds and 13-year-olds crave autonomy, albeit to different degrees; the understanding and skills parents need to navigate the former will prove not only relevant but also valuable in surviving the adolescent years. Similarly, if your toddler's limit testing is making *you* absolutely crazy, as a parent it may be highly worthwhile to explore the intensity of your reactions now, when said limit testing looks like refusal to use a fork rather than refusal to come home for curfew. Your yelling now may lead your toddler to hurl her fork across the floor; your yelling later may lead to something a lot riskier. The point is that the usefulness of the principles explored in this book doesn't have an expiration date. I hope you'll find that what you learn in this book about your toddler's emotions—and your own—will benefit your child's development and the parent–child relationship for years to come.

You may be wondering about whether gender—or, more aptly, biological sex—matters in tantrum behavior. Although research suggests some sex differences with regard to factors that may relate to tantrums (for example, boys typically lag slightly behind girls with regard to language development in the first few years, and tantrums may arise in the context of frustration at an inability to be understood), no gender differences have emerged with regard to tantrums per se, and so the material presented in the book is aimed at parents of both boys and girls.

What We All Need to Know to Deal with Tantrums

This book is organized around four types of knowledge, or building blocks, that we all need to cope effectively with our children's tantrums.

What Is a Tantrum?

It may seem obvious, but, first and foremost, it's important to know what kind of behavior we're talking about. The first two chapters of this book provide this foundation, presenting a useful working definition of a tantrum, discussing the extent to which certain tantrum behaviors are normal, and explaining the different potential functions that tantrums serve. The goal is to learn not only what a tantrum is, exactly, but also to appreciate how the episodes map onto the social and emotional development of young children more broadly.

Why Do Tantrums Occur?

Tantrums don't arise in a vacuum, even though I know it often feels as if your child explodes or melts down completely out of the blue. And so the second building block in our understanding of tantrums is the recognition that they occur within the context of interpersonal interactions; there are unique triggers and family dynamics that precede, surround, and are elicited by them. For example, picture two-year-old Jared throwing a tantrum in the cookie aisle of the supermarket; he's begging his mom to buy the peanut butter sandwich cookies (he's smitten with the bright yellow and red packaging). How would you advise that mother to respond? Do you have your answer? OK, now add to the scenario that Mom is functioning on two hours of sleep, because she has an infant at home, and that—until this very moment—Jared has been a superstar big brother for the past couple of days. Does that information change anything about what you'd recommend? And then what if I told you that Jared's father has a tree nut allergy and that Mom still has bad dreams about the time he ended up in the emergency room after accidentally eating mislabeled Chinese takeout? Or that Mom hates going to the supermarket because it always reminds her of how, as a teenager and the oldest of four sisters, she was the one responsible for doing the family's grocery shopping prior to spending time with her friends on weekends? Or that the family is experiencing financial hardship and is trying to cut down on its grocery budget? Now what?

The point is, we frequently think that a one-size-fits-all approach will work with tantrums, that a concrete set of tools exists to soothe all tantrums the same way a Band-Aid works to protect all skinned knees. In reality, there's no "quick fix." There's no getting around the fact that the context of the tantrum matters. The effort you put toward understanding not only your particular child's stage of development, but also the roles played by you and your family members, is invaluable. Chapters 3–5 get you started on this journey and serve as a guide to piecing together the way that some of these factors may be contributing to your child's meltdowns.

What Can I Do about Tantrums (in Two Simple Words)?

Does all of this mean that, since there's no such thing as a magic bullet, you need to undergo years of therapy before knowing what to do when your son goes completely boneless right before you need to leave the house? Of course not. Enter building block three: the "L words." Decades of developmental psychology research demonstrate that healthy parenting—that is to say, the kind that leads to healthy (and happy, well-adjusted, successful) children—requires the presence of two important qualities: love (the first "L") and limits (the second "L"). Children who thrive feel loved by their parents; they feel seen, heard, and understood, and their homes are characterized by a high degree of warmth. Simultaneously, these children experience their homes as highly structured and predictable, with clear and defined roles and boundaries. That is to say, children need high levels of *both* love *and* limits. The two coexist independently; when one goes down, it doesn't mean that the other goes up, or vice versa. Why is this important when it comes to tantrums? Because tantrums are best prevented and managed when parents deliver these "L words" amply and in equal measure. Once you have a real sense of what that looks like (and you will after reading Chapters 6 and 7), so much else becomes icing on the cake.

Now Please Give Me Some Strategies for the Heat of the Moment!

Yes, finally, you need the true nitty-gritty, the top building block, the deluxe set of concrete behavioral strategies that not only encompass both love and limits but also enable you to cope—in the moment—with the before, during, and after of tantrums. After all, you can accept the normalcy of tantrums, get that toddlers and preschoolers are *supposed* to be controlling, know yourself inside and out, understand that your child's meltdowns remind you of your own father's occasional rage, have a strong sense of the ways in which your spouse's laissez-faire approach to discipline offends your own notion of parenting, be aware of the importance of both love and limits—and yet, if you don't have access to some tools to use right then and there with your little one, there's only so far that these insights, although fundamental, are going to take you. For this reason, the whole second half of the book is devoted to this critical final building block. Its purpose is to equip you with an abundance of practical pointers for tantrum survival, including not only the general *dos* and *don'ts* (Chapters 8 and 9), but also how to apply them at the trickiest times of day (Chapter 10), in the trickiest settings (Chapter 11), and during certain unique circumstances (Chapter 12).

Anything Else?

Throughout the book, you'll find scattered Q&As. These are questions I have been asked repeatedly by parents with whom I've worked, so much so that I wanted to include both the inquiries and my responses in their authentic, entire form. I have a feeling that some of you will have the same questions—or have had these questions asked of you (for example, by a partner, a friend, or your own parents)—and that it will be helpful to have the answers at your disposal as a resource.

Speaking of resources, there is a whole section of them at the end of the book, which I hope you find helpful. Here you'll find books, websites, and other sources of further information and guidance on topics related to tantrums.

Finally, you'll be reading a lot of stories that I hope will strike a familiar chord. In these anecdotes I've done my best to highlight the possible role of different aspects of culture to illustrate that, even though tantrums occur across the boundaries of race, ethnicity, and nationality, of language and geography, of religion and vocation, the particular triggers and responses vary widely from family to family. Please note that these illustrations are all based on actual clinical encounters I have had, although names and identifying details have been changed to protect privacy. Of course, the stories about my own life are presented as is: for better or worse (and likely both!), I am me, Henry is Henry, Zeke is Zeke, and Jon (my husband) is Jon.

How to Get the Most Out of This Book

No matter where you jump in to the material I just described, or how much you get through (because, let's face it, we all have limited time and energy these days), I encourage you to be both open and real with yourself while you read—as I tried to be while I wrote. One of my favorite quotes from the amazing Brené Brown is "Vulnerability is the birthplace of innovation, creativity, and change." My hope is that you will get something of value from this book even if you first thumb through it on a relatively superficial level and skip to the second half for concrete tips to help you get through your day. My sense, however, is that you will get the most out of it if you allow yourself the time and the space—however you can steal it—to wrestle with things a bit, to challenge yourself, and to think deeply about your interactions with your little one(s). Investing time in the first half of the book, in really understanding what's going on with your toddler or preschooler developmentally, as well as within the context of both family dynamics and love and limits, will only enhance the skill and ease with which you're able to implement the strategies discussed in the second half. So even if you can't do so at first, you will get the most out of this book if you read Chapters 1–7 thoroughly at some point. They provide the foundation on which you can build your own set of strategies—those presented in Chapters 8–12, along with the creative solutions you'll be able to come up with yourself as you face whatever your toddler or preschooler throws at you (literally or figuratively) that day (or hour or minute).

Beware Your Assumptions (Tantrums Are Normal!)

I'm just going to say it: this book is not going to cure your child of tantrums. As you'll learn when you are reading this book, and likely know already at least to some extent, tantrums are a normal—and actually healthy—part of development. Toddlers or preschoolers who throw tantrums are learning to express their emotions, assert their independence, forge a place for their needs and wants in what can be a confusing and overwhelming world. This is *not* to say that, as a parent, you just need to grin and bear it. After all, if you came into my basement going on and on about "forging a place for needs and wants" while Henry lay shrieking on the floor about "needing" to watch another episode of *Paw Patrol,* I wouldn't exactly meet you with an easy smile and accepting nod. Don't misunderstand my meaning, though. This book is not going to leave you high and dry, with nothing but a better theoretical, abstract understanding of tantrums. Absolutely not. The book presents what I firmly believe is a practical, helpful framework for thinking about tantrums, as well as a host of concrete prevention and management strategies to learn and implement.

Because tantrums are normal for developing children, and can't (and shouldn't) be eliminated entirely, I deliberately avoid the word "control" throughout the book; please don't look for pointers to "*control* your child's tantrums" (a phrase I so often see in clickbait article titles). Their absence is intentional, because there is no way that we, as parents, can control our children's tantrums—or, frankly, their behavior more generally—any more than we can control anyone else's. Our children are people, albeit little ones—thinking, feeling beings with their own wills, desires, and perspectives—and we need to appreciate them as such. Certainly, there are ways to reduce the frequency and severity of tantrums when they are destroying the family peace, and doing so is valuable for everyone, your toddler included. But "controlling" tantrums, aside from being impossible, is not something to strive for.

Although the words are not perfect, after some struggling, I landed on the idea that, in reading this book, parents will learn to "handle" or "manage" tantrums instead. Semantics aside, my goal is to communicate that, although we cannot dictate our children's ways of being in the world, we *can* take (and not take) certain actions that influence both tantrums and the broader context in which they arise (for example, the parent–child relationship, the home environment).

As you begin to experiment with the prevention and management strategies suggested in the following pages, you'll find that none is a magic wand. Each will work for some children, some of the time. Odds are, you'll find at least one that will work with your particular child most of the time. And that—when it comes to complicated human behavior and relationships—is batting a thousand. Particularly if we're talking about the one-more-episode-of-*Paw-Patrol* tantrum, because, man, that one is a doozy.

Harness the Power of the Pause

Handling or managing (including preventing) tantrums often starts with taking a breath. In fact, to my mind, the most critical goal of the book may be to make it easier for you to put a *pause* between your child's impending or current meltdown and your own reaction. Whether it's because you have a deeper understanding of your child's stage of development, or are more familiar with your own and/or your partner's triggers, or have a toolbox of techniques at your disposal, by the time you finish, my hope is that your response to your child's tantrums will no longer feel out of your control. As a parent, you have choices in how you respond, and the power to make an active versus default choice rests in your ability to take that pause, even if only for a millisecond or two, right before your child takes a vengeful crayon to your living room wall.

Remember That You Know Your Family Best

This book is many things. One thing it is not, however, is the "Hershberg Approach" to toddler tantrums. The book is meant to be a reference, a source of information, perhaps even a comfort, but it is definitely not a bible, or any other prescriptive, be-all-end-all kind of text. This may strike you as a strange thing to say in an introduction, the part where I'm supposed to get you to *want* to read more, to *keep* turning those pages. So why do I say it? First, because life and people and dynamics are complicated; the interactions are not always pretty. There's no way that, in good faith, I can be rigidly prescriptive or guarantee that everything will always work out the way I say it will. What I *can* do throughout the book, and therefore do as much as possible, is illustrate my points with examples of real families—real parents with real little kids who have real tantrums—who use the recommended approaches and tools with mostly positive results. Sometimes I'll even draw on my experience with my own children, not to brag that I've got it all figured out, but, rather, just the opposite—to drive home, time and time again, that this stuff gets messy and that I'm right here getting my hands dirty with you.

A dear friend and colleague recently told me that she feels grateful every single day. What for? In her words: "That when I was doing this work before I had kids, no parent ever told me to eff off." Except she didn't say "eff"; the sentiment merited use of the actual word. On this point, my intention is not to be exclusive. I know some truly excellent child psychologists who don't have kids. I am not saying—and would never say—that you *need* to be a parent to do this kind of work. What being a parent does, however, is remind you *every single day* just how complicated it is, that there's almost never a "right" answer, that the science doesn't always apply to the child, and vice versa.

The science is the second reason I can't support the idea that this book would ever become the "Hershberg Approach." The bulk of what I say is based on wisdom gathered from various fields of study, on theories and evidence-based practices that, in both my professional and personal experience, all coalesce in service of a wise, grounded, and effective approach to handling tantrums. To name only a few examples, the text pays homage to attachment theory, Diana Baumrind's work on parenting styles, and a range of established behavioral approaches (for example, child–parent psychotherapy, parent management training, parent–child interaction therapy). I will gladly take credit for being a discerning and creative curator, but not for reinventing the wheel.

The final reason this book can't ever become the "Hershberg Approach," or the tantrums bible, is that in *your* family, with *your* child, that role belongs to *you and you alone.*

You are the bible, not me. Really. Only you have a deep understanding of your family, with its various cultural orientations, values, and customs. You are in the unique position of being able to adapt the book's many explanations and suggestions to your particular beliefs and standards of behavior. And of course nobody knows your child like you do either: the way that he or she pushes your particular buttons, and how your particular buttons coincide in very specific ways with your partner's particular buttons, which in turn reminds you of your own childhood, which then leads you to respond a certain way to your child, who is right at this very moment banging his head with a spoon.

I'm so excited to be your guide—to point out patterns and commonalities, ways of thinking about tantrums, developmental norms, a bunch of really useful tools, and some not useful and even counterproductive tools. But then I'm excited to empower *you* to put it all together and create your *own* bible of managing your toddler's tantrums. I know it may sound like a daunting task, but we're going to take it one step at a time. Look—you finished the introduction! And that is *not* nothing, given everything else you have on your plate. Now, onward.

"You Haven't Seen a Tantrum Until You've Seen My Toddler's Tantrums"

When Should You Worry?

"You don't understand. Jacob doesn't just tantrum, he completely falls apart. He screams bloody murder. He cries like I'm tearing off a limb; honestly, I'm amazed no one has called the cops! I know you talk to parents about this kind of thing all the time, but I can pretty much promise you that you've never seen any child throw a tantrum the way that Jacob throws a tantrum."

"OK, so I know all about the 'terrible twos,' but this goes so beyond that. My older daughter had some of the terrible twos, and now—I can't believe I'm saying this!—I actually long for those days. What Abigail does goes so far beyond that, it's not even funny. If she doesn't get her way about anything—it could be the smallest, most unimportant thing in the world—she melts down as if the world is ending right then and there."

"The other day, Olivia became so unreasonable when it was time to leave the playground that it was truly a nightmare. I ended up throwing her over my shoulder and carrying her out of the gate, while all these other moms and dads and nannies watched and judged the fact that I couldn't control my own daughter. Or at least it certainly seemed like they were judging. I don't understand: Does every toddler do this? Why does it always seem like it's only mine?"

Each of these quotations is an excerpt from a conversation or email exchange I have had with a parent, and there are hundreds more just like them. When I first hear from or meet parents, more than anything else they want to know whether their child's behavior is normal, expected, part of the typical developmental trajectory. On the one hand, parents want reassurance that, although their child morphs into a Tasmanian devil with some degree of frequency, so does everyone else's. Not only does misery love company, but obviously there is also tremendous relief in learning that your child's behavior is not worrisome per se, no matter how difficult to tolerate. On the other hand, the fact that your two- or three-year-old Tasmanian devil is *yours*—well versed in getting under *your* skin, pushing *your* buttons—often makes the behavior seem far worse to *you* than that of his or her little devil peers. And so the same parents who experience relief at knowing their child's tantrums are typical also don't quite buy it and need their unique experience—that no other devil is quite as devilish as their own little devil—validated. There's weird parent competition everywhere these days. "Oh, you think Lila's pouring milk all over the kitchen floor is bad? That's nothing! Oliver did the same thing but with pee! He seriously took his potty of pee and looked me right in the eye while pouring it on the floor!" And then Lila's mom doesn't know whether to surrender and admit that, yes, urine beats dairy or follow up with the story about the time Lila covered the cat in clay.

Before we go any further, let's define what we mean by normal. For many parents, "normal" is code for "nothing to worry about"; if a child's behavior is normal, then, in colloquial terms, it typically means there is no need for concern—or perhaps even for action. Parents often take comfort in hearing that a behavior is normal because the ensuing assumption is that it will pass with time, that their child will "outgrow" it. And this is certainly often the case with tantrums. What's not the case, however, is that tantrum behaviors are stagnant, existing in a vacuum and impervious to change.

> However "normal" they may be, tantrums can be influenced—and changed—by your response.

Tantrums—even normal, vanilla ones—are influenced by how you, as parents, respond. Therefore, for our purposes, determining whether your child's tantrums are normal is not about rendering parental responses less impactful, but, rather, about figuring out whether a higher level of intervention than that you can offer at home is needed.

Young children begin having tantrums around 18 months of age and continue to do so, to varying degrees, until they are four or five years old, although they generally taper (in frequency, duration, and severity) over time. The episodes typically peak (read: are most miserable to endure) when children are between the ages of two and four years, the age group that's the primary focus of this book. It's probably a relief to know that tantrums as a behavior are normal—in all their soul-crushing glory—during this period of life, but as the parents quoted at the beginning of this chapter can attest, that doesn't mean you're sure that *your* child's tantrums are normal. There are a few different ways to look at the question of when normal becomes atypical or worrisome.

Five *Possible* Red Flags

First, by studying the tantrums of healthy preschoolers compared to those of preschoolers with clinical diagnoses (depression, disruptive behavior disorders), researchers have been able to identify five characteristics, or styles, of tantrums that are considered potential "red flags" for meriting further assessment by a mental health professional:

1. *Aggression toward people or things.* Wait, don't freak out. Some aggression is both normal and expected; as we'll discuss in more detail later on (particularly in Chapter 3), your children are learning to navigate the world and their place in it. Figuring out if and how and where it's effective to express themselves physically is part of this. Not to mention their notorious (and also completely developmentally appropriate) lack of impulse control and response inhibition. In fact, hitting has actually been found to be a common tantrum behavior exhibited by children between 18 months and five years. But if your toddler goes beyond throwing the occasional left hook when you refuse to buy him a candy bar at the drugstore, and is consistently aggressive toward you or another caregiver more than 50% of the time and/or violently destructive toward objects during tantrum episodes, you may have cause for concern.

2. *Self-injury.* Again, take heed—many toddlers or preschoolers may start to bang their head against the wall, or pinch themselves, or hit themselves on the leg when they're upset. And again, this happens for various reasons, not least of all because it's often a surefire way to ensure that Mom or Dad comes running. It's also a behavior that tends to dissipate as children gain more expressive language, as well as prosocial coping skills. But

if a child is repeatedly and forcefully biting herself, scratching herself, or banging her head against the wall or floor, further assessment is likely necessary.

3. *Frequency.* There are days when it seems like all your child does is tantrum. I get it; I really do (no, I *really* do—let's just say that our family spent all day yesterday in an airport and leave it at that). But if your child is genuinely throwing numerous tantrums per day, every day of the week, every day of the month, you may have something to worry about. While I hesitate to provide these exact numbers, lest you open a spreadsheet and go overboard in your tracking, the seminal study that provided the five red flags concluded that those more at risk for a clinical diagnosis had:

- 10–20 discrete tantrum episodes on separate days at home during a 30-day period *or*

- more than five tantrums per day on multiple days during school or outside of the home/school.

4. *Duration.* Sometimes I recommend that parents time their child's tantrums—literally set a timer on their phone when a tantrum begins and stop it when it ends—because when you're in it, a five-minute tantrum can seem as though it's nothing short of three hours. And yes, we can all recall the times when our child's tantrum lasted—actually, truly lasted—a full hour, but that's kind of the point: we remember those times as distinct (and miserable) because they stand out compared to the child's typical meltdown, which lasts somewhere between 30 seconds and five minutes. The same study that found hitting common during tantrums in children one and a half to five years old found that the median length of a tantrum was three minutes, with 75% lasting between 90 seconds and five minutes. Children whose tantrums almost *always* last upwards of 25–30 minutes may have underlying issues that need additional attention.

5. *Inability to self-soothe.* Young children in need of further evaluation and/or intervention typically do not possess the skills to calm themselves down once in the midst of a tantrum. Unless they are removed from the situation, or someone actively helps them, the tantrum behaviors will persist indefinitely. Note, of course, that self-soothing skills are on a developmental continuum and that many young kids need to learn how to take deep breaths, or to count to four, or hug their soothing object of choice before they can implement these techniques on their own.

Clearly, the characteristics on pages 15–16 offer guideposts with regard to whether, and when, to worry about tantrums, and research has continued to bear out the theory that both quantity and quality are important. Looking at a diverse community sample of 1,490 preschoolers, one recent study found that, despite the fact that nearly all children (87.3%) had tantrums sometimes, only approximately 10% had an episode *every single day,* a finding that held across age, gender, and sociodemographic groups. Furthermore, the researchers found that tantrums seem to exist on a continuum, with mild/normative behavior (having a tantrum in the context of frustration or distress, for example) on one end and more problematic or concerning behaviors (such as breaking/destroying objects during a tantrum episode) on the other. Having a tantrum "out of the blue" and having one with nonparental adults were also both indicators of concern, consistent with past research findings in this area.

I know what you're thinking. Your little guy once broke a vase during a tantrum, and it's not like he doesn't ever lose his mind with his grandparents. Once he even fell apart with a babysitter when you took a much-needed night off! And you could swear that he had a tantrum every single day last week, which is what prompted you to start reading this book in the first place. And now I'm telling you there may be something seriously wrong with him? You're about to pick up your phone (if you're not reading on it already) and call your partner, your mom, or your best friend to talk through the evidence . . .

STOP. Deep breath.

Remember Context—and Your ABCs

As stated in the previous section, these characteristics of tantrums are red flags—signs that there *may* be reason to seek a professional opinion. May, may, may! These warning signs are just that; *warning* signs. They are *not* the makings of a precise algorithm for distinguishing worrisome tantrums from more typical ones. Even in the preschool study described at the top of this page, nearly a third of the children in the "healthy" group displayed many of the same atypical tantrum behaviors as their peers with diagnosed emotional/behavior problems, providing evidence that these lines can be blurred or broken. Which is the exact reason I didn't frame them as a checklist of yes or no questions. I can't tell you with precision the specific point at which I become worried, as real children in real life are a lot more complicated than words on a page. Tantrums may be frequent, but not long, or long but not frequent. Clara may hit her mother pretty lightly, but this happens every single time she's upset, and Gabriel, although engaging only rarely in self-injury, may bite himself until the skin breaks. When I evaluate a child's tantrums to determine the level of intervention necessary, I ask about each of these red flags for sure. I also, though, pose many other questions that pertain to both the context and the "ABCs" of tantrums—that is, not only about the behaviors themselves (B), but also about their antecedents (A) and consequences (C).

> Behaviors are much easier to influence when we know what happens before and after them.

"ABC" has its roots in applied behavior analysis, a behavioral therapy intervention (often used with individuals diagnosed with autism spectrum disorder) in which contingent reinforcement is used to increase and/or generalize desired, as well as reduce undesired, behaviors. In plain English, this means that we have the best chance of changing someone's behavior when we don't focus solely on the behavior itself but also know what comes immediately before and immediately after the behavior occurs.

Hugs from Mom *and* a Free Ride on Chores

Roland was a clear example of this. At age two and a half, he was throwing epic tantrums every time his mother asked him to put away his toys. After he screamed and cried for about 10 minutes, his mother would soothe him with hugs and kisses, as well as clean up the toys for him. So in this case, the antecedent, or setting, for the tantrum was the demand to clean up, the behavior was the screaming and crying, and the consequence, or outcome, was Mommy hugs and kisses, coupled with the removal of the demand to clean up.

No wonder Roland was throwing tantrums, right?

I'll talk more about how we determine the causes of, or triggers for, tantrums in Chapter 2, but I mention the ABCs here because they provide necessary context for my assessment of the five red flags described in the previous section. Roland's mother initially told me that he was throwing upwards of 10 tantrums per day and that each lasted more than 15 minutes. Without any additional information, I found her account rather concerning, but I soon found out that Roland was throwing a tantrum every single time his mother made a demand of him, and that each and every time, this behavior resulted in Mommy cuddles and the removal of the demand. With this added information, Roland's behavior became much more understandable—and, frankly, normal. This was not a budding pathology, but rather the natural response of a toddler who had learned a reliable way to get both affection from his mother and his ticket out of an unpleasant task—in one fell swoop! Once I pointed out this pattern to Roland's mother, we were able to work together to change the "C" part of the equation (her response to his tantrums), which in turn led to a change in the tantrum behavior itself.

Bringing Mom and Dad Together with a Tantrum

Here's another example of how key the "ABCs" are, as I want to illustrate this point fully—it's an important one, and we'll come back to it again and again. Serena's mother called to express a concern about the "nonstop tantrum" that her daughter threw every morning at breakfast before preschool. The tantrum, she explained, began the second Serena woke up and continued until she left the house with her father. She would cry, scream, pinch the skin on her hand, and sometimes hit one or both of her parents. As I got to know the family, I learned that the morning was the only time of day during which Serena was home with both of her parents; her father had a demanding job and worked late nearly every night. During my first observation, I witnessed quite a bit of tension between these parents; there was an abundance of eye rolling and some rather hostile tones of voice, in both directions. When Serena was aggressive, however—particularly when she pinched herself—her parents ceased their own bickering and ran to intervene, seemingly in agreement and on the same team for the first time since I'd arrived nearly an hour earlier. Once again, understanding both the setting for and outcome of the tantrum (the antecedent and consequence) was critical. Serena's behavior seemed to be a response to her parents' sparring, one intended (consciously or otherwise) to bring them together. In this case, Serena's self-injurious behavior, while a red flag, was also an understandable, and, again, even normal, response to her family environment. My primary (although not exclusive) recommendation was that Serena's parents work on their own relationship so as to get to a healthier, more connected place. Sure enough, once they did, mornings became more peaceful, and Serena's behavior improved markedly. This is not, of course, to imply that Serena's tantrum behaviors (including pinching herself) were her parents' "fault," but, rather, just that context is key when we attempt to discern whether there's reason for alarm.

"Normal" Is Complicated . . .

I cite these two examples for two reasons. First, I want to highlight the idea that the very question of whether a toddler's tantrums are normal is often a complicated one; not only is the implication of a clear delineation between normal and abnormal misleading, but young children's behavior, no matter how severe or upsetting, can often be considered a "normal" response to particular circumstances. Second, these brief examples illustrate why it would be impossible to establish a formula that determines objectively whether a child's tantrums fall into the majority that are normal or the minority that suggest the potential presence of some pathology.

Does all of this nuance, then, render the red flags useless? No. Absolutely not. There is a reason I included them in this book, and in Chapter 1 no less. Because what these red flags *do* do is offer a *framework* in which to think about the extent to which your child's tantrums are typical and to answer the question of whether it might be helpful to have someone with more expertise—and less bias—weigh in.* After all, as parents, we frequently fall prey to our own version of "medical students' disease," defined by *Wikipedia* as a "condition frequently reported in medical students, who perceive themselves to be experiencing the symptoms of a disease that they are studying. The condition is associated with the fear of contracting the disease in question." Parents read a list of red flags, such as this one, determine—within seconds—that their child clearly meets all of the characteristics described, and promptly hit the panic button.

> Red flags provide a framework, not a formula.

. . . And Also Pretty Common

And so before you go calling your cousin's future mother-in-law, a child psychiatrist who will likely be able to confirm (via text, obviously) that your child, whom she's never met, is indeed a sociopath, please note that there is also some good news. Which is that, from a purely anecdotal standpoint, when parents ask me whether their child's tantrums are normal, *most of the time they are.* As I'll explain in Chapter 2, tantrums are a normal and important part of early child development. So, when parents approach

---

*Toddler humor alert: If read out loud, this sentence suggests the presence of "doo-doo," which is always funny. (I have been in this field for way too long.)

me with concerns that their child's tantrums are unusual or pathological in some way, I generally end up assuring them that this is not the case. This does not mean, however, that I say, "no worries," and send them on their way. Just because tantrums are normal does not mean that they can't, or don't, often cause a great deal of distress for parents. Understanding what tantrums are and how they work—for your particular child in your particular family in your particular home—is important regardless of how "normal" they are. Which, of course, is why I wrote—and you're reading—this book, focused on normal, vanilla, run-of-the-mill (although notably nightmarish in their own right to parents everywhere) tantrums.

When tantrums are normal, they decrease as children get older, their brains develop further, their communication skills improve, and their understanding of the world—and their place in it—becomes more sophisticated. Read: there is a light at the end of the tunnel! That said, we all know older kids—and, frankly, adults—who continue to throw tantrums, even if the behaviors themselves look different. All you have to do is watch the news for five minutes and you'll hear about someone or other—usually a politician!—who, according to the anchor or reporter, is somehow throwing

If, after reading this chapter, you are concerned that your toddler may need a professional evaluation and/or services, the following may be helpful resources:

1. Your local department of health and/or education (in the United States): Many districts offer free early childhood evaluation services, and potentially therapies, for residents.

2. Division 53 of the American Psychological Association, the Society of Clinical Child and Adolescent Psychology, offers a directory of child therapists in the United States and Canada who practice using evidence-based treatments and techniques: *https://sccap53.org/find-a-therapist*.

3. The Society of Clinical Child and Adolescent Psychology provides information about a range of evidence-based child therapy approaches for children, as well as tips for choosing a therapist, at *http://effectivechildtherapy.org*.

The Resources at the back of this book offer more sources of information and help.

a tantrum. So, although a 12-year-old may no longer throw himself on the floor and kick and scream when he is told he has to put the iPad away, he may protest, refuse, sulk, argue, and potentially engage in many more extreme behaviors in response to his feelings of frustration, powerlessness, and disappointment—the very same feelings he had when, as a toddler, he was told he couldn't have more ice cream. This, of course, raises the obvious question: What exactly are tantrums? And how do they happen? These questions will be addressed in the next chapter. As you read ahead, keep in mind that how you, as parents, handle tantrums when your child is two or three years old will have lasting implications for how he or she learns to manage overwhelming feelings—anger, frustration, distress, disappointment, sadness—over time. Because—and this bears emphasizing—*the feelings themselves don't go away.* Our children cease having tantrums not because they become inured to difficult emotions but because they learn to cope with them. How, and how well, they do that is up to you.

"Really? *This* Is What You're Going to Melt Down Over?"

Understanding Causes and Triggers

As an early childhood psychologist, I am asked to give more talks about tantrums than any other topic. When someone from the media requests an article, it's typically one about tantrums. When my mom friends get together, usually at least one person wants to vent about her child's latest breaking-all-the-records tantrum. And yet, even though we all use the same word, we don't always mean the same thing by it. Former Supreme Court justice Potter Stewart famously said in 1964, when attempting to define pornography, "I know it when I see it." And that's how we usually feel about tantrums. That little girl lying on the floor in the middle of aisle seven at Rite-Aid? Tantrum. The little boy being dragged across the train platform by his mother, his empty stroller awkwardly hanging and bumping alongside them? Tantrum. Your precious little munchkin looking at you and shrieking "NOOOOO!" at the top of her lungs right after your in-laws arrive? Tantrum (and, in that case, quite a strategic one, I might add).

But these examples are obvious ones. What about the little girl whose disappointed tears (let's say, over her scoop of ice cream falling off its cone onto the pavement) morph, over the course of a few minutes, into inconsolable wailing? Or the little boy whose fear of thunder results in his covering his ears and screaming, kicking at anyone who tries to calm him down? Are these tantrums too? My guess is that we wouldn't all agree on those—or that, more precisely, we would call them tantrums if we only saw the behaviors in question, but then perhaps backtrack once we discovered their origins. Or would we? Is a tantrum about behavior only, or does the emotion behind the behavior matter too? And if the emotion matters, what about physiological feelings, like hunger or tiredness? Is a tantrum that happens in the context of exhaustion less of a tantrum? Honestly, I don't mean these questions in the philosophical, if-a-tree-falls-in-the-forest sense, but, rather, believe it's important to know what it is we're talking about—especially with something we talk about so darn much. But also because, obviously, the best solutions are designed to address a specific problem. If we don't know what we mean by "tantrum," our responses are likely to be inconsistent and ineffectual.

What Do We Really Mean When We Call Something a "Tantrum"?

I learned early on in my practice that, rather than assuming I knew what a parent meant when she described her toddler or preschooler as having frequent "tantrums," I needed to probe for the actual behaviors involved. Instead of taking the word at face value, I prompt, "Tell me what it looks like when Priscilla has a tantrum." Or, "If I were there, what would I see? What would I hear?" As discussed in the last chapter, I aim to get details not only about the tantrum behaviors themselves, but also about the events that came both before and after, as well as the larger family situation and dynamics. Furthermore, if parents are able and willing, I ask them to guess—with the understanding that there's no way to know for certain— what their child is feeling during typical tantrum episodes.

You might see where I'm headed here: What we mean by the behavior we call a "tantrum" is almost inextricable from the surrounding contextual factors, including precipitating conditions, the problem the toddler may have been attempting to solve, parental/caregiver responses, and all of the emotions involved—for everyone. In my work with families, I've often found that taking into account all of these contextual factors is more important than trying to parse the behavior itself. For example, the literature in this area sometimes refers to the existence of two different kinds of tantrums, those that young children intentionally throw to test limits (to get something they want when they want it) and those that reflect genuine distress and an absence of control over their emotional state. The distinction is emphasized insofar as it dictates the most effective response; children testing limits need firm limits, the theory goes, whereas children in distress need soothing and comfort. Although I would argue that this conceptualization represents a step forward from a one-size-fits-all defini-tion of the term, it still strikes me, from a clinical perspective, as an over-simplification. What we call "tantrums," colloquially and as parents, can emerge in so many different scenarios, escalate in numerous ways, and stem from a range of toddler needs and motivations. Building on Chapter 1, my goal is to provide an accurate, usable definition of "tantrum," but also one that takes into account all of the possible nuances.

Q "I've heard a lot about how some tantrums are kids testing limits, and others are signs of genuine distress. With my kid, though, it's not that clear. He can be totally in control one minute, clearly test-ing his mom and me, and then be having a total meltdown—real tears and all—the next. Is that unusual?"

A No, it's not unusual at all. What you describe is often what young children's tantrums look like, and it's one reason I find that common explanation of tantrums to be—though sometimes helpful on a con-ceptual level—somewhat limiting in helping us respond to real-life kids in real-life situations. A child who is throwing a tantrum—yelling and stomping, say—in the hopes that his behavior will result in your buying him a toy car at the drugstore may seem fully in control of these actions. Until he's not. Once he realizes that the car purchase does not appear to be becoming a reality, he may be overcome with disappointment or frustration and become authentically distressed. At this point, he throws himself on the floor and weeps, which has a genuinely different flavor from the yelling and stomping, yet is still part of the same tantrum. And to make things even more compli-cated? The next day, if a similar situation arises, the tantrum may follow a different trajectory. He may hit that turning point sooner, or later, or not at all, depending on a range of other factors (how tired he is, to use an obvious example). All of which is to say that tantrums, and the emotional states and behaviors within them, can be fluid and complicated. For the most part, it's all par for the course.

Speaking of Oversimplification . . .

Unfortunately, I've discovered that a lot of confusion about the meaning of the word "tantrum" may have originated in some parts of common dic-tionary definitions. Let's start with Merriam-Webster, which defines

> **In this book, what we mean by the behavior called a tantrum has to include:**
>
> - Conditions and events that preceded the tantrum
> - The problem the child may be trying to solve
> - The parent's response
> - The child's emotions
> - The parent's emotions
> - The overall context, including family dynamics, current circumstances, and culture

tantrum as "an uncontrolled expression of childish anger: an angry outburst by a child or by someone who is behaving like a child." Hmmm. This definition didn't completely resonate with me, for a few reasons. First, there's something condescending, in my opinion, about the phrasing. After all, what differentiates "childish anger" from adult anger, from the anger that you or I might experience? Isn't anger a basic emotion, one we all experience, regardless of where we are in the lifespan? Referring to a person's anger as "childish" is, in this context, a way to denigrate or invalidate that person's emotional reaction, even when said person is, in fact, a child. When we think of tantrums as expressions of "childish anger," rather than simply of anger, we are distanced from our little ones, making it more difficult to see the world through their eyes, which is an essential part of understanding (and, thus, helping to shape) their behavior.

> A tantrum isn't just an expression of "childish" emotion (whatever that even means).

Does falling on the floor and screaming because she can't have another cookie constitute an "uncontrolled expression of childish anger" by three-year-old Alisa? Nope, just an uncontrolled expression of regular old anger, I'd say. And actually, perhaps not even that, which leads to another critique of this definition. There are tantrums, as described in the Q&A on the previous page, that *are* controlled. If Alisa knows that falling on the floor and screaming will—at least seven times out of 10—procure her desired second cookie, then over time she may well learn to do this intentionally. At that point, can her tantrum really be called uncontrolled?

Here, however, I need to insert a note of caution: describing a child's tantrums as controlled is not the equivalent of painting him out to be an evil schemer, cackling and rubbing his hands together with a devilish grin as he plans his parents' misery hours in advance. I say this because, all too often, parents will warn, typically with bitterness in their tone, "Oh, he knows *exactly* what he's doing, trust me!" Or, "Wait until you see her theatrics; she is a master manipulator, that one." And then I meet these children, and you know the word that I use to describe them? Smart. These are smart kiddos who have learned to get their needs met in the best way they know how, and—what's most important—in a way that works. In relying on this strategy, they frequently don't develop alternative skills for getting their needs met. Or if they have (say, little Jared is "an absolute angel at school"), then they haven't yet had the experiences at home that would reinforce their use of these skills under this particular set of circumstances. This is very different from a child who has connected the dots in advance and is setting out, in a planned and purposeful way, to get that second cookie by any means necessary. We'll talk more about this when we talk about the specific causes of tantrums later in this chapter.

> Some tantrums are learned (rather than "uncontrolled") behavior, but that doesn't mean your toddler is a manipulative schemer.

Back to Merriam-Webster: Another criticism I have of its definition is that tantrums are not always—and certainly not only—about anger. More often than not, tantrums encapsulate a range of emotions. Children feel angry, sure, but also perhaps frustrated, disappointed, sad, afraid, and/or overwhelmed, to name just a few of the many possibilities. These feelings may be simultaneous or sequential, or a child may go through phases of each. In fact, research involving the analysis of toddlers' vocalizations during tantrums suggests that the experiences of anger and sadness are very much intertwined during these episodes, often manifesting as a discernible rhythm of yelling/screaming interspersed with crying/whimpering.

> During tantrums, children often experience more than one feeling at the same time; check out one of my favorite episodes of **Daniel Tiger's Neighborhood,** "Daniel Feels Two Feelings" (2012).

None of this is meant to point fingers at Webster's dictionaries. The other definitions I found were similarly limited. Dictionary.com, for example, includes the words "violent" and "sudden," and yet parents of toddlers and preschoolers all know that tantrums are by no means always violent and by no means always sudden. So the question remains: What is a tantrum?

Let's review the components we've uncovered—the elements that were found lacking in dictionary definitions:

- A tantrum is not "childish." It's a normal, natural response that is most common in young kids and lessens in frequency as children age and learn more skills for regulating and expressing their emotions (although we all know adults who have shown a propensity to respond this way at times too).

- A tantrum is not always uncontrolled. Sometimes it's a pretty smart adaptation.

- It's not always about anger. Many other emotions—discrete and in combination—can be at the heart of a tantrum.

So, here is a definition that I would offer:

A tantrum is a behavioral response to not knowing how to manage or express an overwhelming emotional experience.

I realize that I've left something out here, because you're probably asking "What *kind* of behavioral response?" We could call it, in a general sense, "acting out," which typically means behaving in some way considered outside acceptable social norms (although it's important to note that said norms are generally based on adult expectations of child conduct, rather than on what we know about child development). That's probably about right. Revisit the descriptions of tantrums at the beginning of Chapter 1 to get examples. I've certainly met parents whose labeling of toddler behavior as a tantrum seemed like an exaggeration to me, sometimes to funny effect, like when they show me a "video of the tantrum" that ends before I think we've gotten to the tantrum part. The fact that these parents recognized, however, that this behavior was an expression of their child's frustration does, however, lead us to an important point: the behavioral characteristics of a tantrum may be less important in defining the term "tantrum" than the role the tantrum is playing for the toddler. Does this mean I'm saying that a tantrum is in the eye of the beholder? As far as the outward behavioral manifestation is concerned, to some extent, yes. Of course if you came to me with complaints about your child's tantrums that, upon exploration, proved to involve whimpering or quietly beating on a toy for a couple minutes, and you revealed an expectation that your two-and-a-half-year-old exhibit the self-control of a 17-year-old, I would strongly suggest you head straight for Chapters 3 and 4 to get a more realistic idea of what toddlers and preschoolers are (and are not) capable of and the ways in which unrealistic expectations can get parents in trouble at these times.

So Why *Does* Your Toddler or Preschooler Have Tantrums?

This past month, I have had several parents ask me, sincerely and with worry in their eyes, if I am absolutely certain that their children are not psychopaths. They ask if I am *absolutely* certain, because they have already asked me on three other occasions. Each time I've offered reassurance that no, their children are not psychopaths; they are just toddlers. My response will float them for a couple of weeks, until their child has another major meltdown, which leads to a repetition of the question: "But wait, are you sure, Dr. Hershberg? Are you really sure she's not a psychopath?"

The question may sound amusing, but none of these parents is remotely amused. (And that's why I decided it was best to get the issue of what's normal and what's not out of the way in Chapter 1.) There is a genuine concern that I couldn't possibly understand the extent of their child's tantrums because psychopathy is the only thing that could conceivably explain the fact that something really seems to be "wrong with her brain." I get it. Just last night, I would have sworn from the pitch of Henry's scream that Zeke had dislocated his arm from the shoulder; alas, Zeke had merely moved Rubble (from *Paw Patrol,* obviously) out of his assigned "parking spot" on the rug. When your toddler comes at you with pudgy fists drawn because you didn't hear his barely audible request that *he* wanted to open the string cheese, it's hard not to believe you are witnessing a criminal in the making.

The (Overly) Simple Answer: Because He's a Toddler or Preschooler

All of that said, when it seems like there's something off in your little one's brain, you're not entirely off base. Young children's brains *are* wired in such a way that tantrums make perfect sense and are actually a sign of normal and healthy development. If adults acted like toddlers in the midst of a tantrum, I might put my odds on psychopathy or psychosis, but when toddlers do so it's a function, at least in large part, of their particular stage of brain development. Which is to say, when we talk about the causes of tantrums, the number-one culprit is—you guessed it—toddlerhood itself. Recent research conducted by Zero to Three and the Bezos Family Foundation illuminated what I see in my practice all the time: parents of children under the age of five consistently overestimate their kiddos' capacity for self-control. Tuning In, the large-scale research effort, is worth checking out, for all kinds of reasons (*www.zerotothree.org/resources/series/tuning-in-parents-of-young-children-tell-us-what-they-think-know-and-need*). In particular, though, the findings highlight what the authors termed the "Expectation Gap," that is, the mismatch between the extent to which parents feel children should be able to control themselves and the extent to which children's young and still-developing brains realistically allow for this control. According to the study, 42% of parents believe that children can regulate their emotions—for example, not have a tantrum in the face of frustration—by age two. In reality, this capacity only begins to develop when children are between three and a half and four years old, and it takes several more years for children to achieve mastery (although, again, keep in mind how many adults you know who could hardly be considered masters of this skill!).

> Our expectations for toddlers' and preschoolers' capacity for self-control are typically far too high.

What Caused *This* Particular Tantrum?

When I share the preceding findings with parents, I frequently see a wave of relief pass over their faces, as it finally sinks in that their child is not, in fact, a psychopath, but rather very much where she is supposed to be along the typical developmental trajectory. But more often than not, that's not the end of the work. If it were, then parents would need only to read an article or two about toddler brain development and all of their fears and frustrations would be allayed. Although toddlers' developmental stage is a huge cause of tantrums, the presence or absence of other contributing factors may increase their frequency, duration, and severity. We can't push fast-forward on this developmental stage (much to the chagrin of some of my clients), but we can play with (a.k.a. work on, but I vastly prefer the former phrasing) these other variables in an attempt to make everyone's life easier.

It's important to know and recognize the more proximal causes of your child's tantrums for two reasons:

1. You're a parent. On balance, it's always nice to understand your kid better and, in this case, to have an explanation for why your house sometimes transforms into the innermost circle of hell and you somehow age 30 years in 30 minutes.

> "Toddlerhood" may well be the answer to the question of why your child is having tantrums in a general sense, but that doesn't mean there aren't concrete and important reasons that your child had a tantrum yesterday afternoon.

2. As we've established, the more we understand about a particular tantrum—including figuring out patterns and trends—the more effectively we can prevent their occurrence and/or intervene appropriately.

A Quick Note on the Word "Cause"

Any of you who have ever taken a social science class can probably still hear your professor harping on the point that "correlation does not equal causation." That is to say, the fact that two things are related does not necessarily mean that one caused the other. Take heart attacks and baldness; many people who have heart attacks are also bald, which is to say, heart attacks and baldness are highly correlated. If I shave my head, however, do I increase my chances of having a heart attack? Of course not; despite their *correlation,* baldness is not the *cause* of heart attacks. Another example would be if you had a headache, took some ibuprofen, and your headache got worse. Would that mean the medicine caused the headache to get worse or was a *trigger* for the worsening headache? Well, we happen to know (or, at least, assume, barring very unusual circumstances) that this is not the case, because we know at least a few things about headaches and we know at least a few things about ibuprofen. One could imagine, however, that someone who didn't know these things might make that assumption, given the order in which the events occurred—that is, that the medicine came before, or was a *precursor* to, the more painful headache. A precursor, or an *antecedent,* is merely that—something that comes before another thing in time.

When we talk about tantrums, the words "antecedent" and "precursor" are the most technically accurate; we can never say for certain that something *caused* or *triggered* a tantrum per se, because there is no way to prove it. For example, do I know beyond a shadow of a doubt that exhaustion was the cause of Henry's *Paw Patrol* meltdown last night? Of course not; I can't do a blood test to demonstrate that or redo the evening with him less tired to see whether the meltdown would still occur. It would undoubtedly be more accurate to say that exhaustion was a precursor to— or, even more precisely, a preexisting condition for—the tantrum. As someone with a research background, I still believe strongly in the importance of being precise with our language and meaning, areas in which sloppiness and misunderstandings can have disastrous effects (read: the antivaccination movement). And yet, as a mom, I feel comfortable saying that *of course* exhaustion was one of the causes of Henry's tantrum yesterday. Because when we talk about the causes of tantrums in this book, we are speaking colloquially, not scientifically. I'm also doing my best to avoid jargon, because, well, no one likes a jargon-talker.

Triggers, Causes, Antecedents: It's Possible (Likely) That a Lot Is Going On at the Same Time

Keep in mind that there can be more than one factor operating at the same time, and in different ways. So, for example, let's say that Isaiah's parents tell him that he needs to turn off the TV, immediately prompting a tantrum. Most immediately, it seems that wanting, and not being able, to watch more TV is the trigger for his yelling and crying. And it clearly is. But then, let's say that it's 5:00 P.M., and Isaiah hasn't eaten since he had lunch at 11:30 in the morning. In that case, hunger would be a probable trigger as well. And then let's add to the scenario that Isaiah's family just moved to a new house and this is his first night there (Mom and Dad were on the ball and got the TV hooked up before they actually moved in—huge props to them!). Well, then, the new environment, with all of its ensuing emotions, is likely a trigger—or backdrop—as well. And so, when we think about how to intervene with this tantrum, we need to keep in mind all three triggers— a task that becomes even more important if we want to *prevent* another tantrum the following day.

Behavioral psychologists understand the idea of multiple factors involved in bringing on a particular event (in this case, a tantrum) so well that they've come up with what is called a behavioral chain analysis.* It shows that any behavior follows from a set of linked factors, from conditions that increase vulnerability to the behavior (Isaiah's hunger making him more easily frustrated than he'd usually be by being told he can't keep watching TV) to significant events that have an impact that lasts for a while (the move to a new house) to more immediate triggers (the TV being turned off). All of these add up to an overflow of frustration, and—boom—a tantrum that seems to (but doesn't) come out of nowhere. If you feel like it, think of your child's most recent tantrum and fill out the form on page 34 to list the links in the behavioral chain that might have led to the meltdown.

What's the point of reliving this particular nightmare? It helps you see that more might have been going on than you thought. But it also illustrates a really important underlying point about behavioral chain analyses: Any link in the chain offers an opportunity to head off or intervene in a tantrum. Until you get to Chapter 8 in this book, almost everything you'll read is about how to understand the backdrop causes of tantrums and what you can do to prevent tantrums by applying that understanding. Once you get to Chapter 8, you'll find a wealth (really) of strategies you can use to deescalate a tantrum once it's already started, followed by some ideas for preventing tantrums at times of day that are ripe for meltdowns, anticipating troublesome environments (that is, places that seem virtually designed to set off your toddler), and managing in circumstances that are particularly challenging for developing little minds and bodies.

Despite the many links that can make up the chain for an individual child, there are some issues that are so frequently and commonly associated with tantrums that they are worth delving into in more detail.

Common Causes of Tantrums

Although the causes of tantrums (again, above and beyond the developmental norm and expectations) are many and varied, there are a few common categories that account for the majority.

Being Tired and/or Hungry

Undoubtedly, sleep and food are two biological needs that every toddler—nay, every human has. Toddlers—nay, humans—are a mess when they

---

*The behavioral chain analysis is an important tool in dialectical behavior therapy; both the tool and the therapy were originated and developed by Marsha Linehan.

Links in the Chain That Led to Today's Tantrum	
How was my child feeling before the tantrum? (Tired, hungry, sick, already frustrated, sad . . . ?)	
How did my child sleep last night?	
Any big changes in my child's world in recent days or weeks?	
How did the day go overall? (Smoothly, with lots of little hassles, nothing went right . . . ?)	
How were my mood and stress level today?	
How were my child and I getting along today?	
Were we interacting with anyone else prior to the tantrum? How might this person (or persons) have contributed somehow?	
How was I feeling right before the tantrum?	
Did I have any expectations about how I wanted my child to behave that may have been unrealistic?	
What happened right before the tantrum?	

are tired and hungry. Period. Sleep is one of the very first things I assess when I speak with new clients who have sought my help with tantrums. If a toddler is not getting enough sleep, I always suggest we start with getting sleep back on track before we delve too deeply into any other point of intervention. And sometimes that's all it takes. If you are struggling with your toddler's tantrums, do yourself a favor and look at his or her eating and sleep patterns, as it may be that a few adjustments in these realms will make a world of difference. If, in so doing, you determine that these need to be your area of focus before you read any further, please see the Resources at the end of the book.

One more note on this. I recently worked with a father who commented how funny it is that little kids don't know when they're hungry, that they rely on adults to decode the feeling for them. His remark came on the heels of an episode during which he had to physically put food in front of Christopher, his three-year-old, despite Christopher's repeated protests that he wasn't hungry (uttered during what his father termed "multiple mini-tantrums" at the playground). Of course, once Christopher saw the string cheese, Goldfish, and cut-up apple in plain sight, he essentially inhaled it all in three minutes flat and proceeded to be in a much cheerier mood for the rest of the afternoon. I'll remind you to think about food and sleep in the strategies for preventing and intervening in tantrums throughout the rest of the book.

His comment got me thinking, though: Is it only toddlers and preschoolers who don't recognize their hunger, or are adults sometimes guilty of this as well? I know that I've certainly had days when I feel grouchy, and when I stop to think for a moment, I realize that I haven't eaten anything yet, or that I had a particularly small breakfast or lunch. Often, once our hunger or tiredness has affected our moods, we no longer realize that they are the culprits. In this way, we're not so different from our little ones. Picture yourself when you're hungry and sleep deprived, except minus the coping skills and self-awareness you've had years to develop. Bingo. Let's let them off the hook a bit. Chapter 4 will go into detail on our own role in triggering tantrums.

Environmental Events and Transitions

This is a bit of a catchall category, and I'm not sure how to avoid that. Essentially, it includes a host of "events" (for lack of a better word) that shake little kids' worlds and around which they experience a lot of emotion. When toddlers and preschoolers have big feelings, they often get overwhelmed, which may, for some children, look like acting out, or tantrums. These events include (but are not limited to):

- A new sibling
- Moving
- A change in caregiver (including the end of a preschool year and transition to camp, or vice versa)
- Parental separation/divorce
- Some kind of trauma (car accident, medical procedure, exposure to violence, death of a loved one, etc.)

This book will not focus at all on this latter category (trauma), about which much can be said and has already been written (see the Resources should you be in need of guidance in this area). Seeking the help/guidance of a professional is frequently recommended in these cases. It does, however, bear emphasis here that, for young children, tantrums can be the manifestation of a range of emotions and are not limited to an expression of frustration or disappointment. Within the context of trauma, they may signify confusion, overwhelm, grief, anger, shock, anxiety, or any combination thereof.

In the case of the more ordinary life events (those that many families experience at one time or another), the concepts and strategies outlined in this book will still be helpful, potentially in addition to other more targeted interventions. You can implement the tools discussed here and supplement with other resources aimed at helping toddlers and preschoolers digest a particular event, such as moving or the birth of a sibling. I offer some specific ideas in Chapter 12.

Expressive and/or Receptive Language Problems

Children with language delays frequently display an increase in the frequency and/or severity of their tantrums. As you can imagine, it can be extremely frustrating to have a lot to say (and how much there is to say when the whole world is brand new!) and not be able to say it. It can be equally frustrating—or confusing, or demoralizing, or upsetting—to know someone is trying to communicate with you but not to understand his or her meaning. In both cases, in addition to their immediate frustration, children may feel shame or isolation, as if there is a barrier separating them from others. Not surprisingly, therefore, research has shown a high

correlation between language and behavior issues in children. If you sus-
pect that your child's tantrums may be related to an issue with language
expression (speaking) or reception (understanding), talk to your pediatrician about the best way to have your child evaluated for delays in this area.
I have worked with many families who report a significant improvement
in their child's tantrums once speech therapy is under way and some language gains have been made.

Parenting That Inadvertently Reinforces Tantrums

Yup, you read that correctly. You can close this book now because, at the
end of the day, it's all *totally your fault*. OK, I'm kidding with that last line.
Sometimes I make a joke like that with parents in my office, and I see even
the most laid-back, good-humored mom look wounded for a moment before
she gets that I'm kidding. We need to laugh at how quickly we assume the
worst in ourselves, at our immediate assumption that somehow we may
unknowingly be doing something that is slowly but surely ruining our children before our very eyes. Please remember: none of this is about blaming.
Rather, it's about understanding. Certain types of parenting are more likely
to lead to tantrums than others; we need to be able to talk about this without sinking down into a giant shame spiral, recognizing that we're all doing
the best we can to raise our little alien creatures—er, I mean toddlers, and,
uh, preschoolers.

In my practice, there are primarily two ways in which I see parenting
lead to increased tantrums.

Inconsistent Limits

The first is when parents unintentionally reinforce, or reward, tantrums
by either giving in to the request at hand or giving the behavior a great
deal of attention—attention that the child would not otherwise receive.
For example, let's say that Ella and her mother are at the drugstore. Mom
accidentally walks Ella down the packaged candy aisle (cue the soundtrack
to *Jaws*), and Ella (of course) demands a candy bar. When Mom denies her
request, Ella begins to melt down—screaming, crying, the works. At her
wit's end, Mom finally gives in, exasperatedly mutters, "fine," and thrusts
a candy bar at Ella, who promptly quiets down as she begins to unwrap
her coveted treat. In this case, Ella's mother has taught Ella a valuable lesson and one she will come to regret. Namely: tantrums work! Think about
it:

- Ella asks for candy, Mom says no, Ella is quiet = no candy.

  versus

- Ella asks for candy, Mom says no, Ella throws a tantrum = candy.

Are there times when we need to give in to a tantrum? Of course. But over time, if you give in most of the time, or even more than occasionally, your kiddos will learn that throwing a tantrum is an effective way to get what they want, or, at the very least, that it works once in a while and so it's worth a shot. In addition, even if you stay strong and don't give in per se, you can still reward a tantrum with your focus and attention. Let's go back to the drugstore with Ella and her mother, and this time let's say that Mom doesn't ultimately give Ella the candy she's demanding. Instead, let's say that she continues to say no, to explain to Ella why she can't have candy (explanations may range from the fact that sugar is bad for her teeth to the fact that she had candy the day before, to the price of the candy, etc.), to implore Ella—for the love of all things sacred—to be quiet, and, finally, to do all of the above while picking her up and carrying her (perhaps even leaving the store). In this case, Ella learns the same lesson, because although her tantrum hasn't been effective in getting her the candy she wants, it *has* worked to get her something even more valuable, that is, the singular focus and nonstop attention of Mom. And, as anyone with a toddler knows, that's nothing less than solid gold right there. To break this one down:

> If what a toddler wants is attention from you, and that's what every tantrum produces, how many tantrums is the child likely to throw? (No, I didn't say there would be math, but this is a rhetorical question.)

- Ella asks for candy, Mom says no, Ella is quiet = Mom focuses on getting what she needs at the drugstore, maybe spends a bit of time checking her smartphone, perhaps pays some attention to a sibling.

  versus

- Ella asks for candy, Mom says no, Ella throws a tantrum = Ella gets ALL MOM ALL THE TIME.

In this way, put simply, rewarding tantrums with either the thing in question (candy, another TV show, etc.) or merely an abundance of attention will ultimately lead to more tantrums over time. Showing (and, thus, teaching) your child that tantrums are *not* the way to get what you want—whether that be a particular thing or attention from

Mom or Dad—is the way to reverse this pattern, and Chapter 8 goes into detail about some of the specific strategies you can use to do this.

Neglecting to Validate Your Toddler's Emotions

The other way that parenting can lead to increased, or more severe, tantrums occurs when parents continually neglect (or forget, or refuse) to validate their children's emotional experiences. Let's go back to your favorite place—the drugstore—with your favorite company, Ella and her mother. Once again, Ella's mother ends up with Ella in the candy aisle (when will she learn?). Ella, as has become the custom, begins to have a meltdown after her mother refuses to get her the candy for which she is flat-out begging. Except in this version of the example, Ella's mom neither gives in and gets her the candy nor continues to pay Ella a great deal of attention while she continues to scream and cry. No, in this case, Ella's mom belittles, or invalidates, how Ella is feeling, remarking that not getting candy is "no big deal" and that Ella needs to stop with the "water works." And so now Ella needs to cry harder and scream louder because her mom just isn't getting it—it's as if she's countering: it *is* a big deal, Mom, and these tears are completely warranted, so there! Ella may have originally been crying about the candy, but now she's even more upset because she doesn't feel heard or understood by the person who's supposed to be in her corner. Moreover, she may even feel ashamed of the big feelings she's having, as Mom made clear they are not appropriate to the situation. Of note, this will likely be the case even if Mom's comments are expressed in a kind, rather than biting, tone, or with a sympathetic smile, as in "Ella, sweetie, relax; you sound like you're being tortured!"

In my experience, invalidating children's emotional experiences is an extremely common way that parents accidentally amp up their children's tantrums. Furthermore, this is often done with the very best of intentions—parents regularly tell me they want their kids to have a "thicker skin" or to "not get upset over every little thing." And yet, paradoxically, in their efforts to "toughen up" their toddlers or preschoolers, they end up sending the message that they don't understand or care about their little ones' feelings, which only serves to make these feelings—and the corresponding crying, yelling, and kicking—stronger. Which is not to say this goal—of building children's resilience—is not a worthy one. After all, we all want nothing more for our kids than that they be able to overcome the hardships they encounter, and we know that having to forgo candy at the drugstore is nothing compared to the obstacles that lie ahead for them as adults. And yet, downplaying or negating the strong emotions to which toddlers and preschoolers are prone is not the way to get there. Rather, we foster resilience both by teaching and showing our children *how* to handle difficult feelings and by voicing support and confidence in their ability to do so.

> Resilience is built not by protecting our kids from their strong emotions but by helping them learn to handle their feelings and supporting them in doing so.

Q **"Does my child always need to 'feel heard'? Sometimes he's going to need to tough it out! I don't want to raise a snowflake!"**

A I hear some version of this question at least once a week. Parents recognize that the world is not always a loving, validating place and want to make sure their little ones are prepared for—and can handle—that reality when the time comes. They wonder whether empathizing with, or validating, children's feelings too much will somehow make them "soft" or more vulnerable to the many obstacles that will undoubtedly crop up on their path. I always respond with a few key points.

First, keep in mind that you are validating *feelings, not behavior.* Your child has a right to feel however she feels, in part because—no matter how much we may want to—we can't control another person's (even our child's!) emotional experience. We can, however, and should, provide guidance about the behaviors that are and are not acceptable in response to certain feelings. As you'll learn as you read this book, validating emotions never needs to come at the expense of setting limits, and, if it does, then nobody wins.

Second, one of your jobs as a parent is to "right-size" feelings, which is different from invalidating them. If your child is losing his mind because there's a speck of something you can't even see on his french fry, then the idea is to say something like "It seems like you're really not happy that your french fry doesn't look exactly the way you want it to." In this way, you're providing language for her experience and applying a calmness and simplicity to what likely feels like a very overwhelming experience for her. This differs in important ways from, say, "You are absolutely falling apart about the tater tot! Sweetie, are you OK? This is so overwhelming!" The latter, while descriptive, does nothing to soothe your child or communicate your confidence in her ability to handle the situation.

Which leads to the third and most important point. All the research shows that the way to develop resilience, or "toughness," in our kids is by ensuring they feel confidence in their own coping abilities. How do we do that? Not by teaching them to distrust or undervalue what they feel, but rather by showing them that feelings—though difficult—are manageable. When children are young, they need to know that their parents and caregivers are on their team, rooting for them. It is only with that knowledge, that felt sense, that they can meet their full potential and take the world by storm. If they sense that you may or may not be there for them, may or may not really see who they are, may or may not value their experiences as legit, they'll never have the confidence they need to be the not-a-snowflake you know they can be!

Naming Ella's feelings for her and connecting them to the event at hand (thereby creating a narrative out of what may feel like a giant ball of emotional chaos) is a way to do this: "I see how upset you are. You're feeling frustrated and disappointed that you can't have candy right now, huh? You really, *really* want that candy." For more concrete examples of how to add this important tool of validating emotions to your toolbox, again, please see Chapter 8. Also see Chapter 6, where I explain the concept of rupture and repair within the "love" part of "love and limits," the foundation of tantrum damage control. (Hint: When you yield to the strong instinct we all have to tell someone whose distress is distressing to us that the person shouldn't be upset, thus invalidating the person's emotional experience, that's a rupture. When ruptures happen in our relationships with our children—which they will, and quite often!—we need to do a repair so as to keep the parent–child relationship authentic, strong, and healthy.)

Because we, as parents, can control the ways in which we parent on a day-to-day basis (at least most of the time!), the bulk of this book focuses on this last category of tantrum causes—that is, how parents may unintentionally increase tantrum frequency or severity by interacting with and reacting to their toddlers or preschoolers in certain ways.

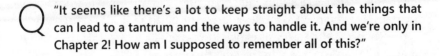

Q "It seems like there's a lot to keep straight about the things that can lead to a tantrum and the ways to handle it. And we're only in Chapter 2! How am I supposed to remember all of this?"

This is another conversation I have with my clients quite regularly. A lot of this is new information, and—depending on your own background and situation—like learning a whole new foreign language. Which it's impossible to do overnight. And yet, if you immerse yourself in a new language, and make efforts to practice it, and are gentle on yourself when you make mistakes and speak imperfectly, then slowly, over time, you develop a mastery. You begin to speak the language less self-consciously, more naturally, fluently. That's what this is like. Yes, there's a lot of information to take in. And yes, we all want instant gratification, and a lot of us feel bad about ourselves when things don't click right away. I'm currently in a rather lousy mood because I clearly didn't do a good job pumping air into my tires this morning, because the stupid tire pressure light is still on, as if mocking my total incompetence—and I have taken this as a measure of my self-worth despite not exactly aspiring to be a naturally gifted *auto mechanic*. If I can go down that shame spiral after a quick stop at a gas station, trust me, I can imagine where you go when it comes to feeling bad about your parenting your toddler. Go easy on yourself. Really. You'll get there. Even just reading this far is a huge step.

When it comes to looking at the causes (or triggers, antecedents, contexts) of tantrums, it's important not to go down a rabbit hole. I could write pages more about why toddlers and preschoolers have tantrums, and, in fact, a father named Jason Good beat me to it, when he penned a list in 2012, titled "46 Reasons My Three Year Old Might be Freaking Out." I laughed out loud when I first read the items included, and continue to do so to this day. Classics include "His lip tastes salty," "A balloon he got six months ago is missing," "His brother looked at him," and "His brother didn't look at him" (*http://jasongood.net/365/2012/12/46-reasons-why-my-three-year-old-might-be-freaking-out*). Just to remind yourself of how charmingly funny your child's tantrums are, you might try writing your own list of things that have been known to freak him or her out. I have done my best, though, to list what I have noted in my experience to be the major categories of reasons toddlers and preschoolers tantrum—in addition, again, to the fact that they're toddlers and preschoolers—with the goal of helping you diagnose what's going on with *your* child, in *your* home. Because only by understanding and exploring the likely triggers for your child's tantrums can you begin to think about the steps that you need to take to address the tantrum situation head-on.

A good place to start this exploration is with a look inside the toddler brain, and then your own, in the next two chapters.

3

"What's Going On in That Curious Little Mind?"

Being Realistic about the Limitations of the Developing Brain

DAVID: Mommy, I want a toy. Can I get a toy?

MOMMY: No, honey. We're here to get a birthday present for Sammy.

DAVID: But I want one!

MOMMY: Honey, it's not your birthday; it's Sammy's birthday.

DAVID: (*louder and more upset*) Please???

MOMMY: David, stop. I said no.

DAVID: (*yelling*) I WANT A TOOOOY!

MOMMY: David, are we going to have to go home?

DAVID: (*Starts crying.*)

MOMMY: David, why are you crying? You have so many toys at home! You just got so many new ones for Hanukkah. Come on, now. Stop crying and act like a big boy.

DAVID: (*Keeps crying, looks down at his shoes.*)

This interaction took place at a toy store in Manhattan a couple of years ago. I had stopped in to buy my nephew a birthday present and overheard the exchange as I waited in line. I don't know for certain how the conversation ended, as at that point I paid for my build-it-yourself ninja robot spaceship and left the store. I would be willing to bet, however, that David got increasingly upset, while his mother got increasingly frustrated, and that the combination resulted in an all-out meltdown—definitely on David's part, and likely on his mother's too.

We can't talk about tantrums, and different approaches and strategies for decreasing their frequency and intensity, without spending some time talking about the little culprits—toddlers and preschoolers—themselves. After all, as discussed in Chapter 2, toddlerhood itself is the leading cause of tantrums everywhere! That is to say, it is the nature of the young brain that underlies many of the various causes of tantrums we just reviewed. Tantrums don't make sense (read: they often seem full-on bonkers insane) without a deeper understanding of toddlers and preschoolers more generally—what they can and cannot do at this particular stage of development, the ways in which they see the world, and how they conceptualize their place within it. As parents, when we don't have this understanding, we—just like David's mother at the toy store—unintentionally pour fuel on our children's simmering meltdowns in our heroic efforts to do just the opposite.

Although toddlerhood is generally defined as 12–36 months, in this chapter I'm zeroing in primarily on two- and three-year-olds, as that's typically when families contact me for help with managing their child's tantrums. Certainly, the behaviors can emerge as young as 12 months (and occasionally even younger), but they don't blossom, so to speak—really, truly flourish (!)—until a bit later. And on the other end of the spectrum, don't be fooled into thinking that tantrums will cease the minute your child has his fifth birthday. Although many of the behaviors do tend to decrease around this time from a purely developmental standpoint, there are plenty of reasons they frequently persist well into the preschool and even early school years.

So what exactly is going on in the brain during this stage of development? Certainly, there are numerous resources (some listed at the end of this book) that delve into this critical topic in a much more thorough and nuanced way. For our purposes, however, a mere rudimentary sense of what abilities are already developed, what abilities are in the process of developing, and what abilities have yet to develop—specifically toward the capacity to avoid having a tantrum—will go a long way toward furthering our understanding of what's happening (and not happening) when our little ones are sprawled across the floor, kicking and wailing like it's their job (which it is).

A Work in Progress: The Toddler Brain

On a very general note, let's pause and clarify exactly what we mean when we talk about "brain development." Our brains are made up of billions of neural connections that fire across different areas of the brain; these connections become the neural pathways that ultimately comprise different brain structures, or our *brain architecture*. Neural connections fire at very high speeds in early childhood—more than one million new connections are formed every second in the first few years of life—during which time there is also a vast increase in brain volume; a brand-new infant's brain is 25% the size of an adult's, then increases to 80% by age three and 90% by age five. Neural connections are then decreased through a process of *pruning*, which results in fewer, but more efficient, neural pathways, or circuits, as we grow. To that end, we can also look at brain development as a function of the *speed* of neural processing, which increases exponentially as our circuitry becomes more efficient (and so faster) across infancy and childhood. Brains are built in a given order from the bottom up, with simpler pathways (hearing and vision, for example) developing first, followed by those of increasing complexity.

The ability *not* to have a tantrum necessitates, not surprisingly, neural circuitry that is quite complex, requiring an interrelated collection of social, emotional, and cognitive skills. Specifically, when we look at tantrums, we need to look at the capacities children have to perceive the world around them, regulate their emotions, communicate and use language, problem-solve, and use various executive functioning skills, such as those needed to exercise judgment and make decisions. These abilities exist in several areas of the brain—including the prefrontal cortex, limbic cortex, basal forebrain, amygdala, hypothalamus, and brainstem—all of which are structures that undergo a period of rapid development in the first few years of life.

The Feeling Brain versus the Thinking Brain

When tantrums seem to be characterized by uncontrollable emotions, one of the distress systems—related to rage, fear, and/or separation—has likely been activated. The areas of the brain responsible for these reactions are fully developed from birth, as, from an evolutionary standpoint, they are necessary for survival. These responses reside in a baby's lower brain and are activated so often in the first few months of life because the higher brain—where rational thinking and problem-solving skills are located—is far less developed. As babies enter toddlerhood, areas of the higher brain develop further, which allows for more capacity to override some of these more primitive responses. However, the pathways between the lower and higher brain remain inefficient, such that—put extremely simply—emotions can't always "talk to," and therefore be soothed by, rational thought. These are the tantrums my clients describe as "a switch flipping" in their child, or as their child's "being hijacked" by the strength of her reaction.

> Toddlers and preschoolers are in the process of mastering a number of emotional, cognitive, and social skills that allow them to have fewer tantrums as they grow.

And so, when we look at children between the ages of two and four, whose brains are developing along a typical path, we can think about two simultaneous phenomena. First, when we compare four-year-olds to two-year-olds, we see some mastery of various emotional, cognitive, and social skills that allow them *not* to have tantrums where their younger counterparts do. Second, we also see that ongoing development in the upper brain, as well as the neural circuitry between the upper and lower brains, results in tantrums that continue to occur with some regularity.

The Growing Capacity *Not* to Have a Tantrum

Let's take a closer look at David. Although he ultimately fell apart when his mother wouldn't let him get a toy, he demonstrated some crucial skills before that happened. First, David did not simply reach up and grab a toy that he wanted. It's easy to take that for granted, but, if David were a baby, he wouldn't have been able to stop himself! Now, however, he has a few things going for him that help him out. For example, he has the *working memory* capacity to remember certain rules; he knows, and seems to remember in the moment, that he is not permitted to simply grab things off shelves in stores and take them just because he wants them. He also has the *inhibitory control* to override his desire to do this, let alone, potentially, to hit or otherwise be physically aggressive toward anyone who gets in his way (in this case, his mother). This is an important executive functioning skill that begins to develop in early childhood and that, again, we don't see in younger children, who reach out and grab anything that looks enticing (read: small things they can put in their mouths).

Once it's clear that David is able to refrain from grabbing the toys, we begin to see some of his *expressive language skills*; he is able to ask his mother in simple and clear words for a toy and to express that he really (*really!*) wants one. He even says please, suggesting an understanding of manners and, possibly, conversational norms. Note, also, his *receptive language skills*; he clearly understands his mother's responses—variations of "no"—which is presumably why he becomes more and more upset.

If we shift and look at David's internal experience (or, rather, what we can assume it to be), it's clear that he has a certain level of *awareness* about how he feels; he sees something that he wants and knows he wants it. He also seems to be aware of his mother's emotions, as his level of upset corresponds not only to her words but to her facial expressions and seemingly exasperated and frustrated manner as well. Furthermore, when David's mother prompts him to act like a "big boy," David looks down at his shoes, suggesting that he feels shame in that moment; this is a somewhat complex feeling, in that it requires a sense of self in relation to others. In contrast, telling babies to act like big kids is relatively futile, because the abstract thinking involved (implied, hypothetical comparison to others) is not yet present, and, relatedly, neither are these more nuanced emotions.

All of these skills—working memory, inhibitory control, expressive and receptive language, emotional awareness of self and others, experience of complex emotions—are interrelated and, in this example, came together to help David *not* have a tantrum at the toy store. Until, of course, he does. Because, although he has these skills in varying degrees, he doesn't have them fully, and it is just as easy (and often easier) to view the example through the lens of David's deficits. Be honest: When you read the dialogue that opened this chapter, did you see a child who successfully managed *not* to have a tantrum for a couple of long minutes due to his amazing cognitive, language, and emotional capacities? I didn't think so. I imagine that, instead, you saw a child who wasn't able to regulate his emotions and impulses and who fell apart when he didn't get what he wanted after a few short minutes.

The latter perspective is not wrong—at all. There is no question that, the same way David *was* able to inhibit some of his impulses in this scenario, he wasn't able to inhibit others (for example, yelling). And the same way he *was* able to understand and use language in certain ways, these skills were also limited; it's likely he didn't understand what it's not being his birthday had to do with his wanting a toy, and simultaneously wasn't able to express his confusion. We often think about how frustrated *we* feel when toddlers and preschoolers can't express themselves (or when we can't understand their attempts to do so), but imagine how frustrating this must be for *them*! Think about it: Have you ever heard a toddler say, "Hold on; I'm confused. Can you please break that down for me?" Didn't think so. But does that mean toddlers don't experience confusion? Of course not. There is a lot about being a toddler that is quite confusing; Mom's explanation that you can't have a toy because it's not your birthday is just the tip of the iceberg. Finally, although David was aware of some of his internal experience—namely, his desire for a toy—he was likely unaware of much as well, including, say, that he was hungry, or tired, or felt disconnected from his mother. Self-awareness is also a work in progress and sometimes even eludes adults, as we've already noted and go into further elsewhere in this book.

The Toddler Brain on Overdrive

We often don't recognize that our toddlers are working so hard, in an ongoing and nearly constant way, *not* to have a tantrum, and that this task alone takes an extraordinary level of energy, effort, and skill. Which, as an aside, is one reason that tantrums increase, in both frequency and severity, when toddlers are tired or hungry. In those moments, they just don't have the reserves required to expend energy on keeping it together. Think about how hard David's little brain was working in those few moments alone—and then imagine that, hypothetically, he had accompanied his mother to Rite-Aid minutes earlier, where he didn't have a tantrum after his mother denied him a candy bar at the checkout counter. His little brain has been on overdrive!

Appreciating Your Young Child's Mental Efforts

As parents, it's our job to see toddlers' and preschoolers' ongoing, and often unspoken, efforts to make sense of their world—internal and external—as the astonishing feats of strength they are. And yet, it's a job that most of us aren't that good at; we're much better at noticing, and often becoming frustrated by, the ways in which their social, emotional, and cognitive skills are lagging. David's mother is pretty quick to dismiss not only David's request for a toy, but also his ensuing emotions; she sees them, at best, as an inconvenience and, at worst, as a personal slight. The next chapter, which focuses on who *parents* are in the common interactions leading up to and during tantrums, will do a deeper dive into the specifics of what may be going on for her. On a general note, though, it's clear that she, at least in this moment—like all of us, much of the time—doesn't necessarily grasp where David is developmentally and how his behavior is perfectly in keeping with what we'd expect it to be.

The more we can take into account the ways in which toddlers' brain architecture and neural circuitry both have and have not developed—because both things are true—the more we can understand that a good portion of their behavior stems from this, rather than, say, deliberate vengefulness and/or budding sociopathy. And when, in turn, we simply *expect* certain behaviors, we feel less angry when those behaviors—our kiddos shrieking in public, or taking a crayon to the wall, or denying taking and eating the cookie that you *just watched them take and eat*—occur. Or, at least that's the way it'll work on most days. On other days, who cares about their stupid brains because OMG he just took a crayon to our newly painted walls!

Five Characteristics That Fuel Toddler Tantrums

The remainder of this chapter focuses on remedying this common disconnect that exists between parents and toddlers or preschoolers, as I've experienced it in my work with clients. (And never, ever as a mother. Ahem. Sorry, just clearing my throat.) Specifically, I elaborate on five characteristics that most toddlers have in common and that emerge as a function of their developmental stage: *impulsivity, rigidity, emotionality, a need for control,* and *egocentrism*. I chose to underscore these five qualities in particular because, in my experience, they are both the ones that help explain, in broad terms, the bulk of typical tantrums and are also the ones many parents tend to misinterpret or misunderstand—often inadvertently making tantrum behaviors worse. For my clients, learning that these five qualities are both normal and expected, as well as more about how they play out in daily life, often leads to a profound sense of relief. And once that relief is there, the stage is set for a deeper understanding of their child, an ensuing sense of compassion and connectedness, and the space to interrupt the "tantrum rut" and explore new and different ways of responding.

1. Toddlers and Preschoolers Are Impulsive

As referenced earlier with regard to David's inhibitory control, young children's executive functioning skills—namely, a collection of abilities related, among other things, to self-control and mental flexibility—are barely developed. The Harvard Center on the Developing Child compares the human brain to an airport and this important set of capacities to a sophisticated air traffic control system that handles the numerous arrivals and departures of many different planes on several different runways. Executive functioning develops well into a person's twenties, which means, to run with the analogy, that our little ones are without a doubt flying planes this way and that, banging them into each other, changing their destinations without warning, and, essentially, in a state of perpetual disorganization. Occasionally, one plane may get where it was scheduled to go, but that's often the exception rather than the rule. What does this look like in a real-life child (who, thankfully for all our sakes, is not actually running an airport)? With self-control and mental flexibility absent (in two-year-olds) or barely present (in four-year-olds), you see a great deal of the opposite, namely impulsivity and rigidity. First, let's explore the former.

Take Tommy. You may tell Tommy five different times and in five different ways on the walk to the playground that he has to wait his turn to go on the slide, knowing that this has been a problem in the past. And Tommy may agree, nodding earnestly in complete agreement, perhaps even furrowing his brow in disapproval of his past tendencies. And when you get to the playground, Tommy may still drop your hand like a hot potato and beeline as fast as he can for the slide, immediately cutting ahead of the line and racing up the ladder. "Are you *kidding* me?" you think to yourself (or perhaps say out loud), followed by a shout: "Tommy, we *just* talked about this! You *cannot* cut ahead like that! You *said* you understood!" And the thing is, he did understand. And—even more maddeningly—probably still does! But Tommy's understanding is no match for his impulsivity, and that's what took over once the slide was in plain view. And because you don't necessarily think about this in the moment, you do what so many of my clients do: you pull Tommy aside (once he's down the slide), and you pose the $65,000 question: "Why did you just do that?" Tommy may stare at you blankly, or shrug, or look away; I don't know Tommy, so I can't say for sure. I can, however, assure you that he does not have a satisfactory answer to your question. Because one does not exist.

Because toddlers are often ruled by their impulses, they don't always plan their next move—they just make it. And because grown-ups don't operate this way—and we are often truly puzzled by the choices our toddlers make ("Really? You're eating the Oreo you just dipped in the leftover ketchup?")—we ask them to share their thought process. And they can't. And we get frustrated, because we really do want to understand. And they get frustrated too, because they really, truly can't answer. Sometimes when I do observations in my clients' homes, I keep track of how often parents begin their sentences with the word "why" during their children's meltdowns:

"*Why* are you crying?"

"*Why* are you acting like this?"

"*Why* did you just do that?"

"*Why* are you ignoring me?"

I keep waiting to meet the four-year-old who answers, "I'm glad you asked, Dad; I'm acting like this for a few reasons, including that I'm frustrated, I don't feel understood, I'd really like you to give me what I want, I'm trying to make a point, and I'm four and can't help it." But it has yet to happen. Go figure.

Think about it—how many adults do you know who could answer these questions in the heat of the moment? Sure, maybe a little later, after emotions have died down, some reflective and thoughtful conversation might occur, but while tempers are running high? Unlikely. This is because, even as grown-ups, when our emotions are activated, they often "hijack" our executive functioning skills (see: road rage). And so, even when they're not mid-tantrum, toddlers typically can't answer these questions. Just last week, I had the following conversation with Henry at the dinner table, after he suddenly and seemingly for no reason threw a piece of tomato-sauce-covered tortellini across the kitchen, immediately prompting me to forget everything I know about toddler brain development:

DR. HERSHBERG, RENOWNED EARLY CHILDHOOD PSYCHOLOGIST (!): Henry, why on earth did you just do that?

HENRY: (*Blank stare, bit of an impish grin.*)

DR. H., R.E.C.P.: No really; why?

HENRY: (*Shrugs.*)

DR. H., R.E.C.P.: (*this time, louder and slower, for emphasis*): Henry, why on earth did you just take a piece of tortellini off of your plate and throw it across the room like that?

HENRY: *(cheery smile, as if this is totally obvious)* Because I did.

Needless to say, that cleared it all up for me. Sigh. No doubt, in airports without air traffic control systems, it's important to beware of sudden and unexpected flying pasta.

Seriously, though, asking little kids why they do what they do, or feel what they feel, or act how they act, just doesn't really get you anywhere. At this age, they are generally not going to provide satisfying answers, not only because their cognitive and language skills are not up to the task, but also because often a reason doesn't exist. Aside from, of course, the important fact that the toddler brain is, at times, programmed in such a way that it reverses the famous adage and leads kids to "do before they think." A quick note, however: Do you see the word "generally" in the second sentence of this paragraph? Note that word. And think back to David at the toy store, before he had a meltdown, when he was able to control his impulses. Because toddlers' executive functioning skills are in the (long) process of developing, their emergence is not predictable beyond certain generalities. There are countless moments in a day when your toddler *is* controlling her impulses, when she doesn't hit even though she feels like it, or waits to cross the street until you take her hand, and these moments increase in frequency as she grows. It's just that, as parents, it's so easy not to notice these moments—especially compared to those when you're getting slugged in the thigh or watching your child dart into oncoming traffic, both of which are hard to miss.

Let's go back to the playground. The day after Tommy cuts ahead in line, he tells you over breakfast that he wants to go back to the slide, because he now knows how to wait in line. You're skeptical, but sure enough, when you get to the playground, he walks over to the slide, looks at you and grins, and takes his rightful place behind the other children. He waits patiently, then goes down the slide, then runs over to you for a giant hug. He is clearly so proud of himself! And, for that matter, you're pretty proud of yourself too! Such a great moment, such a swelling heart, a sigh of relief that the days of playground embarrassment and yanking Tommy away from the slide are, at long last, behind you. Except they're not; the very next day (so, for those keeping track, day three of our playground series), Tommy resorts to cutting in line once more. And you are so frustrated, maybe even livid. *What gives?*

The toddler brain for the win once more. These skills develop over time, and, though they certainly trend in the right direction (if all is going smoothly), the journey is not a linear one, and so it's far from predictable. In general, two-year-olds have way less control over their impulses than four-year-olds if we take a longitudinal and broad perspective. But if we take just one two-year-old and one four-year-old, at just one moment in time, then the differences between them in this area may be harder to see. And that's true with all of the characteristics described in this chapter. Although most toddlers embody these qualities at some point, they do so to differing degrees and at different times, depending on a range of factors, including temperament, biological/genetic makeup, and surrounding environment. An awareness of where young children are in their brain development roughly between ages two and four provides a helpful context for acquiring a deeper understanding of their tantrums. It does not, however, account for the variation that of course exists. If you are a parent to more than one child, you know exactly what I'm talking about.

> Remember that toddler development, while mostly proceeding forward, is not linear and therefore can be unpredictable.

2. Toddlers and Preschoolers Are Rigid

And now, the latter manifestation of no air traffic control system: rigidity. Young children are learning to make sense of the world around them, which can often seem big, overwhelming, and unmanageable. In the absence of skills that allow for mental flexibility, their attempts to bring order to chaos often come across as rule-bound and unyielding—or, in the words of many of my clients, absurd and ridiculous. Repetitive behavior, rituals, and ceremonies around daily routines are all extremely commonplace in young children and an important way that they start to make sense of their surrounding environment. This is simultaneously completely normal and thoroughly maddening.

I recently spoke with a father who, along with his family, lives on the 12th floor of an apartment building. Somewhere along the line, his daughter, Serena, had decided that she needed to count to 12 every time they were about to ride in the elevator—before they actually pushed the button calling it to their floor. This was problematic for three related reasons. First, like many parent–toddler teams, Serena and her father were typically in a hurry on most mornings. Second, like many toddlers, Serena was not known for her speed counting and, rather, had an extraordinary ability to turn even single-syllable numbers into multisyllabic recitations (wuh-uh-uuhn; twooo-ooo-oooh; three-eeee-eee). Third, if Serena's father attempted to push the elevator button prior to Serena's getting to 12, a full-on meltdown would inevitably ensue and then continue until Serena was permitted to get to 12 prior to the elevator's arrival (that is, it didn't "count"—no pun intended—if the elevator had already arrived). Serena's father was convinced, as parents who reach out to me often are, that his daughter had the beginnings of what was sure to become obsessive–compulsive disorder.

Nope. After asking a few important diagnostic questions, I determined that, instead, Serena was just a typical ritual-obsessed toddler, wreaking havoc on her parents' sanity (and schedules) the way ritual-obsessed toddlers often do. Which is not to say that this particular behavior stemmed only from her rigidity around ritual per se; many of the characteristics of this developmental stage are overlapping, and so it's likely that a desire to exert control over the situation (described in detail later in this chapter) also played an important role. But her parents had humored her for a few days when she initially did the counting before the elevator thing (they thought it was cute), and so, soon enough, she had come to rely on the ritual as an important part of the morning routine. The lesson? Never underestimate the tenacity with which toddlers will cling to "sameness" or predictability as a way to manage their worlds. As parents, we need to both understand and accept this facet of our children's behavior, so that when the time comes, we can put limits on it, as well as manage the inevitably ensuing tantrums, more effectively.

Along similar lines, many tantrums stem from things not being "just right" in our toddlers' opinions (and—of course—what is just right can vary from day to day, given toddlers' infamous emotionality, also described later in this chapter). In the past month alone, clients have listed the following as reasons for their children's meltdowns, all of which I would put under the heading "I wanted things to be an exact certain way, and you either didn't read my mind or accidentally totally messed things up":

Mommy put Joey's fork on the plate instead of next to Joey's plate.

Baby Jess bumped into Ella's line of cars, knocking one out of its place.

Daddy put two ice cubes in Michelle's water when she only wanted one.

The lights were on when the family got home, when usually they're off.

Mommy took a different route to day care to avoid traffic.

Mommy's shirt was tucked in the wrong way.

Someone plugged the nightlight in to a different outlet.

The noodles were a different shape than usual.

The booster seat was upside down when Marco got to the table.

You get the idea—and likely could make your own list. The next time you think to yourself, or complain to a friend, that your little one "gets upset about the littlest thing"—words I hear daily from parents—do your best to remember this aspect of toddlerhood. To you these things are little. If an adult were upset about the placement of a fork on the table (let alone lying on the floor and shrieking about it), the sight would be very worrisome indeed. To toddlers, however, these things can be big. Their little brains are working so hard to make sense of their world, and mental flexibility—sometimes this thing happens this way, and sometimes this thing happens that way, and sometimes this thing happens that other way, and all are OK—is a skill they are just beginning to develop.

Of course, you can't be expected to predict each thing that's going to set your toddler off or to prevent the subsequent upset. I've seen parents who try to do this, and it's a fast road to Crazytown, as well as a potentially harmful message to communicate to kids (that is, that you, or they, can't handle their reactions). What you *can* do, though, is expect and accept that your little ones are going to be hyper-observant at this stage; they are going to watch you like hawks, and notice everything you do, in their ongoing quest to figure out all they can about how things, and people, work. If you skip a page of their favorite book (by accident or because it'll bring you two minutes closer to bedtime, not that you're counting)? They'll notice. If you pronounce the fruit that grows on trees in Florida as "ore-range" instead of "ahr-range" one day? They'll ask why. If you tell them the story about when they were born but leave out the thing you said last time about how Daddy was so excited? They'll call you on it. And then, when they ask you, eagerly, how Daddy was feeling, and you say he was happy? Well, then, they'll sulk, and turn away from you, because that's not what you said last time.

While we're on sulking . . .

3. Toddlers and Preschoolers Are Ruled by Emotion, Not Logic

Considering the realities of brain development, it should come as no surprise that, nine times out of 10, your toddler operates from a place of *feeling* rather than *thinking*. When David is at the toy store, the fact that he *wants* a toy is sufficient enough reason, in his mind, that he should to be able to *get* a toy, and no logical explanation in the world is going to convince him otherwise. Not only that, but the two explanations his mother uses—that he has so many toys at home and that he just got so many new toys over the holidays—are bound to fall completely flat. By definition, being ruled by emotion means that toddlers live in this moment and this moment only; unlike adults, they can't (and therefore don't) reflect on the past or plan for (or worry about) the future. If David's limbic system (a.k.a., the "emotional" brain) were more articulate, it might respond, "Why are you bringing up this completely irrelevant what-I-have-at-home business? Right now, we are at the toy store, and I want a toy right here, right now!"

> Trying to get an emotional toddler to see reason is like speaking louder and louder to someone who has told you he doesn't speak the language.

And, if David's limbic system were on a roll, it might go on to note, "I know I got a lot of toys for Hanukkah, silly! That was awesome! Which is why I want more toys! What part of this don't you understand, Mom?"

The Perils of Trying to Reason with a Toddler or Preschooler

So often, my clients attempt to rationalize with their little kids, then feel frustrated when they are met with blank stares, defiance, or tantrums. In these cases, it's as if parents and children are speaking different languages—and the misunderstanding goes in both directions. Toddlers don't have the capacity to grasp the logical explanations put forth by their parents, and parents frequently don't get just how intensely their toddlers feel. Continuing to rationalize with a toddler is like repeating your words louder and slower even after the person to whom you're speaking has made it clear that she doesn't speak the language. Here are some examples that come up a lot in my practice.

Brushing Teeth. Toddlers are notorious for not wanting to do this. Why? Because they don't feel like it. Because, objectively speaking (with apologies in advance if you are one of the rare few who feel otherwise), brushing one's teeth is not particularly interesting or enjoyable. Necessary? Yes. A good time? Not so much. And, for many kiddos, no Disney-character toothbrush or watermelon-flavored toothpaste is going to change that. Parents, on the other hand, are notorious for attempting to speak to their little ones about dental hygiene; I've had clients who have actually used the words "halitosis" and "gingivitis" while chasing their two-year-olds around the house. Want to guess how that worked out for everyone?

Dawdling. Synonyms provided by Google include *linger, dally, take one's time, be slow, waste time,* and *idle.* The only one missing? TODDLER. Because when they're not running around like little road runners, they're frequently moving reaaaaaallllly slowly. Why? More to the point: Why not? To little, constantly exploring brains, the world is a fascinating place; what could possibly be the reason to do anything or go anywhere quickly (excluding scenarios involving cookies, cake, or ice cream, of course)? And what are silly grown-ups constantly trying to do? You guessed it. Explain—with carefully considered logic—why it's important to move faster. Said rationale frequently involves a discussion of what time it is, words like "late," and phrases like "they're expecting us" or "it starts at." Concepts that mean nothing to toddlers and preschoolers and that pale in importance compared to the thing on the rug over there under the couch that no one else can see but that's apparently a little bit sparkly.

Touching Fragile Objects. I once worked with parents who complained that their little girl was constantly throwing tantrums because she wasn't allowed to touch the very fragile—and shiny and gorgeous—glass vases that were on display in her living room, just out of her reach. Her parents' ongoing explanations that the vases were delicate and easily breakable did not seem to deter this little girl's argument—that she really, really, REALLY *wanted* to hold them—in the slightest. And round and round they'd go.

It's not that you should excise all logic from your interactions with your little ones; providing rational explanations to your kids can be a helpful teaching tool, depending on both content and timing. I think we would all agree that, for example, a short and clear explanation about why it's important to hold a grown-up's hand to cross the street (for example, "Cars come fast and I need to be able to pick you up if one comes too fast") is both helpful and important to include in a conversation about expectations for taking walks in the neighborhood. It is *not*, however, an effective way to calm your toddler down *after* she has jumped off the curb by herself, you have grabbed her wrist, and she is in the midst of screaming and crying as though you have broken both her arm and her spirit for today as well as all of eternity.

What *will* work in that moment? You'll find lots of ideas in Chapters 8–12. As a general rule, though, think about how you would communicate with someone who didn't—and couldn't, at least right now—speak your language. You'd have no other choice but to learn his. For toddlers, this is, first and foremost, the language of emotions, of desires.

What else is going on for the little child who wants to run into the street all by herself, or who wants to choose when to brush her teeth (never), take her time in leaving for preschool, or pick up the century-old crystal bowl bequeathed to you by Great-aunt Millie? I'd be willing to bet that this child is, at least on some level, attempting to assert her control. Because, though I'm not generally a betting woman, young children's need for control is pretty much something you can always count on.

4. Toddlers and Preschoolers Are Seeking Autonomy and Control

As our little ones are learning about the world around them, they strive to achieve independence, or autonomy within it, and to have more control over their day-to-day experience. No longer content to give themselves wholly and naively over to the wants and needs of the grown-ups, they now want a say in how things go. And often that's not quite enough; what they actually want is the *ultimate* say in how things go—to be the boss, run the show. And yet (thankfully!) because the grown-ups in question are still actually in charge, we continue to tell our toddlers and preschoolers what to do, pretty much all of the time—when to leave the house, when to sleep, when to put on their shoes, when to change into pajamas, when they need to use the toilet or be changed, when they can have screen time, when they can have a snack. And when we're not telling them what *to* do, we're telling them what *not* to do—don't touch that, don't go over there, don't talk to me like that, don't hit your sister, don't put that there, stop yelling, stop whining, and so on. So much of what we, as parents, say on a given day is a direct challenge to our toddler's desire to be more autonomous. No wonder conflict—and the potential for a tantrum—waits around every corner!

I can't tell you how many times parents sit in my office, shaking their heads incredulously: "Honestly, sometimes it seems like he actually enjoys not doing what I ask him to do, like, takes genuine pleasure in it!" My response: "Right. Because he DOES." Or they observe aloud, "It's like she cares about disagreeing with me more than she cares about absolutely anything; if I say black, she'll say white, but if I then change my mind and say white, she'll say black!" Again: "Yup. Sounds about right." Or my favorite, "It's like he has fun saying no—he says it before I even finish my sentence, before he even knows what I'm asking him to do!" Once more, "Yes. A million times YES."

Each of these parents is picking up on something very real, and critical to remember when thinking about tantrums. In a choice between exerting their autonomy and almost anything else (again, cake perhaps excepted), young children will nearly always choose autonomy. If you make it clear that you are invested in Thing A (say, their taking a bath), they will make it even more clear that they are invested in the opposite, or Thing B (not taking a bath). If you then capitulate fiercely and insist they don't take a bath, they may well beeline for the bathroom and start getting undressed. Of course, for the latter to occur, they'd have to really buy in to your capitulation—toddlers are both smart and tuned in, which can be a deadly combination when it comes to sniffing out inauthenticity. Although "reverse psychology" tactics can be effective with these miniature control freaks (because, come on, let's call them what they are), it can be even more helpful to hold your true desires (in this case, your child's cleanliness) a bit closer to the vest and/or to build in opportunities for them to exercise actual control. More on this in Chapter 8.

It's during my conversations with parents about their toddlers' need for autonomy and control that I frequently hear about the most epic tantrums:

> "Who does he think he is? The only person who has ever had to do anything he didn't want to do?"

> "I look at her, and I think to myself, 'You don't know how good you have it.' I mean, I wonder how she'd act if I were making her do something that was genuinely unpleasant. I just want her to clean up her toys, for crying out loud!"

> "Sometimes, I just need him to do what he needs to do, period, end of story. I don't have time for this. He is not the center of the universe."

Ding ding ding. There's nothing like a battle over something seemingly (read: to adults) small to remind us that a lot of the time toddlers and preschoolers do actually believe they are at the very epicenter of existence, with all else—including their parents—revolving around them. This characteristic is termed egocentricity; it's a big one, and it's the final one discussed in our exploration of developing brains.

Before we go into egocentricity in more depth, however, let's stop for a moment and think about how the ways we've described toddlers and preschoolers thus far—as generally impulsive, rigid, emotional, and control/autonomy-seeking—can interact and/or appear in combination. Let's take Tyler. Tyler is almost three, and he's obsessed with rocket ships. He loves nothing more than lining up the various rockets he has in size order and playing "space." He tells his mother exactly what her role in the game is, including that she is not "allowed" to help him count down from 10 to 1 (even though he can't yet do so himself), but does "have to say 'blast-off' in a loud voice" when he points at her (controlling, rigid). If the game doesn't go exactly as he describes, he screams and gets upset (rigid, emotional). One day, as he is playing with his mother, his 17-month-old sister comes over and grabs one of the rockets out of its rightful place in the line; Tyler screams "Noooo!" at the top of his lungs and smacks her on the arm, despite the well-established rule of no hitting (emotional, impulsive). He is then absolutely inconsolable for the next several minutes, noting, as tears stream down his face, that his sister "messed up the whole game" and that she must return the rocket to its place on the line "right now" so that he can start the game from the beginning (emotional, rigid, controlling).

When Tyler's mother described this scenario to me, she actually paused at this point in the story. "I mean, what did he *think* was going to happen?" She asked me, incredulously. "Did he think Lucy [his sister] was just going to let him line the rockets up like that without somehow getting in the way? Did he forget that she was there?" Both good questions if you don't have a solid grasp of toddler development. In response to the first, it's not that Tyler thought his sister would act in a certain way or not; rather, it's that he just didn't think about it at all. Having that kind of forethought, let alone adjusting his behavior accordingly, would involve both planning and higher-order problem-solving skills, neither of which is in place at his stage of development. Tyler was living in the moment, plowing forward without really thinking ahead, as toddlers do. In response to the second—whether Tyler forgot Lucy was present in the room—it's hard to say. What's not hard to say, however, is that toddlers are self-focused; particularly when they're highly involved in an engaging activity, they don't have the ability to see the situation at hand from another's perspective. Lining up the rockets was all about Tyler's own enjoyment and desire, and it would have been beyond his mental capacity to realize in the moment how enticing the line would be to his baby sister. In short, Tyler was being egocentric.

5. Toddlers and Preschoolers Are Egocentric (and, at Times, Unempathetic)

In short, what egocentrism means is that young children believe the world revolves around them; they're notoriously unable to see the world from another's perspective. When David walks in to the toy store with his mom and sees all the toys on the shelf, chances are he believes they are there for his own personal enjoyment; after all, *why else would they be there*? And so, prior to any words being spoken, David and his mother have different—and opposing—views of the task at hand. David's mother knows the goal is to purchase a birthday present for Sammy, and David's pretty sure that the goal has something to do with him and his present-moment experience, because, well, what else is there? When David says he wants a toy and his mother counters with the actual purpose of the errand (purchasing a gift for Sammy's birthday), her response may not make sense to him. I've heard children, depending on personality and age, ask things like "But why isn't it my birthday?" Or, "Can we make it my birthday?" or declare, begging for consideration, "But I *want* it to be *my* birthday!" From their perspective, these responses are completely reasonable: "It seems like you're telling me this outing is not about me, which is not at all to my liking. But since you seem to be stuck on that, here are some adjustments we could make!"

No wonder it sometimes seems like parents and toddlers/preschoolers are already butting heads merely upon walking in to a stimulating setting. And, of course, a "stimulating setting" doesn't have to be a toy store or the candy aisle of a supermarket. It can also mean, for example, the sidewalk, where suddenly your little one becomes fascinated by the shape of the cracks in the cement ("Mommy, they're like snakes!"), particularly, it seems, on the mornings that you're already running late to work. Your attempt to put an end to the sidewalk marveling by explaining your boss's expectation of punctuality is likely not going to be an effective strategy in this case, and moreover may yield defiance and/or a tantrum. Why? For a few key reasons.

First and most fundamental, as discussed earlier, young children don't have any real sense of time to begin with, and so the concept of "lateness" is going to go right over their little heads. Second, though, why else would the cracks exist in the sidewalk if not to be studied intently? How puzzling that you don't seem to care about them! Can't you just look a little harder? Your toddler is certain that if you just take a minute to look closely, your mind will undoubtedly be blown by their reptilian likeness. Because his is. And if his is, yours must be too. Finally, egocentrism dictates that—in her mind—your child's needs and desires trump everything else, all the time. You may need to get to work on time, but your child is feeling curious, and so of course that's her—and should be everyone else's—priority.

Within this context, the concept of empathy often comes up with parents. After all, when toddlers and preschoolers act as though they are, and rightfully should be, the center of the—and, more specifically, *your*—world, it's easy to feel resentful. Think about the last time you were attempting to do 122 different things at the same time when your toddler asked you for something, then immediately burst into tears when you hadn't dropped everything to rush to his side within three seconds. In that moment, your toddler is experiencing the ultimate injustice: he has a need, and, for a reason he truly—literally—cannot wrap his brain around, you are not making it your number-one priority. You, though, in contrast, feel almost insulted when he begins to cry and blurts out, "Can't you see that I'm doing something?! I'll be there in a minute!" The next chapter will explore the different ways in which our toddlers' tantrums can trigger our own emotions (in this case, say, feeling unseen or unappreciated, neither of which is his responsibility). The answer to the immediate question, however, is yes and no. Your toddler can, of course, see that you are doing something, but, because he is, by definition, all about himself, he doesn't understand why this would (or even could) get in the way of whatever is on his agenda. He's not really looking at you, or thinking about you, other than in relation to *his* experience and *his* needs. Is he a budding narcissist with no capacity for empathy? Highly unlikely. He's just a young child with completely developmentally appropriate egocentrism.

As it happens, empathy—the ability to feel or imagine someone else's emotional experience—is a complex skill set that develops throughout early childhood. There are actually thought to be two different kinds of empathy—emotional and cognitive—that have different developmental trajectories. Emotional empathy refers to the ability to feel how someone else is feeling, the vicarious experience of another person's emotional state. Research has shown that signs of this quality can be seen as early as infancy, and it emerges by age two in most toddlers, as evidenced by the demonstration of helping behaviors (offering comfort/advice, attempting to distract) to someone they perceive as distressed. When I talk to parents about emotional contagion—your baby picks up on how you are feeling!—it is this quality that I reference. Cognitive empathy is a bit different, however, and refers to perspective taking, or the ability to imagine another's experience. Cognitive empathy emerges later, only around age four or five years.

This disparity—between the emergence of emotional versus cognitive empathy—is highly relevant to the example on the previous page. Your toddler *does* see you are doing something, and may even understand—or vicariously feel in that moment—that you are frustrated. That does not mean, however, that he grasps why. He cannot yet put himself in your shoes and perceive that his need—no matter how urgent to him—looks quite different from your perspective. Imagine how confusing or frustrating this could be. Think back to David at the toy store. He gets that his mother is exasperated and getting angrier, but is unable to comprehend exactly why, because he is not yet able to see the situation through her eyes. She, meanwhile, sees that he is registering her exasperation and can't understand why this isn't leading him to change his behavior—to stop asking for a toy, or to stop crying.

Meeting Young Children Where They Are

Toddlers are toddlers. Preschoolers are preschoolers. Which is to say they are all, on some level, impulsive, rigid, emotional, yearning for autonomy and control, and egocentric—less than when they were babies, and more than they will be when they're kindergartners. As little kids, they are right on track. It is not your child's job to see the world from your perspective. Their little brains don't yet have that capacity. Ours, however, do—what a gift when we use it! When we take these different qualities into account and see the world through our toddlers' eyes, suddenly so much of what they throw tantrums about makes sense ("sense" defined loosely, of course). And, at the same time, so much of what we say in our attempts to calm them down does not.

It might take a little practice—or at least a pause and a step back—to meet our little kids where they live, developmentally speaking, and understand what's going on with their tantrums. To take that step, consider doing a little exercise along the lines of how I characterized Tyler's behavior when his little sister "ruined" his space game. Write down the story of your toddler's last tantrum. Then take a look at each aspect of your description and see if you can label the developmentally normal characteristics manifested—impulsivity, rigidity, emotionality, the need for control, and egocentrism. It just might make you look back on the event differently, as well as help you reframe future tantrums this way while they're happening.

Young kids have one job and one job only: to be young kids. When your little one pitches a fit because his water is too wet (as I saw in a comedian's tweet the other day), he is doing *exactly what he is supposed to be doing*. And if you are expecting anything different—like, say, that your toddler act like a school-age child—that is on you. Your little one's brain can only do what it can do, and it's up to you to accommodate to that. Notice I didn't say accommodate to *your child*; I am not advocating for an approach that gives in to every one of his whims and wishes. What I *am* advocating for is an understanding of what your little one can and cannot do at this stage and a willingness both to accept and to work within those parameters.

The thing about parenthood is that it's not a balanced relationship. If you make some changes to how you act or react, chances are it will change the nature of your interactions with your child, but those changes need to start with you, not with the child. There is a wonderful saying, used in a variety of contexts, that it is important in human interactions to "be the thermostat and not the thermometer." I don't know whether the original author (whose identity I don't know) had parents and young children in mind, but the words could not be more relevant. Your toddlers are, and will continue to be, at least to some extent and for a little while, egocentric, emotional, impulsive, rigid, and controlling. In common parlance, that means that they are going to be real pains a lot of the time. Of course, they're also going to be silly, adorable, hilarious, insightful, and sweet—but these characteristics don't often show themselves during tantrums, which is our focus. They will be all of these things because they are little. And now, armed with this knowledge, you have the opportunity to adjust your actions and reactions accordingly.

Q "My three-year-old genuinely seems to believe that everyone else wants, thinks, and feels the same things he does. No matter how many times we explain that different people want different things—like, he may want to go to the playground right this second, but Mom and Mommy need to relax for a little while—he doesn't seem to get it. It's beyond frustrating—for him and for us. What should we do?"

A The first thing I am going to do is correct the first sentence of this question by omitting the word "seems." Why? Because your three-year-old doesn't just *seem* to believe that everyone shares his beliefs, desires, and intentions—he full-on *does* believe this. Which puts his brain exactly where it's supposed to be at age three. And so my first response to your question of what to do is quite simple: wait. It's not until between the ages of four and five that children develop what's called "theory of mind"—the ability to understand that other people have their own unique perspectives, and that it is *their* thoughts, feelings, beliefs, and intentions that guide their behavior, rather than either yours or some objective reality. Ever been on the phone—the old-fashioned, non–FaceTime kind—with a young child? You ask him, say, what he ate—or even what he's currently in the process of eating—for dinner, and there's a deafening silence, right? Now, of course, this can happen for a few reasons—he's distracted, he doesn't have sufficient expressive language to respond, etcetera. But he may also be baffled because don't you know what he's having for dinner? Can't you see from where you are? Doesn't everyone know, and see, what he's having for dinner? It sounds nutty to us adults, but this is how children think before they've developed theory of mind.

There have been a ton of studies looking at how and when this capacity develops, many of which use what are called "false belief" tasks. For example, let's say you present a young child with a box of Teddy Grahams. You open the box and show her that, instead of delicious little bear-shaped cookies, inside are actually baby carrots. You then close up the box and pose a question to the child: "Maria has never seen this box of Teddy Grahams. What will Maria think is in the box, cookies or carrots?" If the child has developed theory of mind, she will be able to understand that Maria will lack knowledge about the reality of what's in the box, and so will have a *false belief* that it contains, as would be suggested by the outside of the box, Teddy Grahams. Maria, therefore, will have a different perspective than she does. If the child has not yet developed this ability, then the answer will, of course, be carrots; she knows carrots are in the box—and carrots *are*, in fact, in the box—and so Maria will of course know this too.

My second response to your question is to note that, despite there being a clear developmental trajectory along which theory of mind develops, there are certain things you can do to help promote this ability. Namely, talk about other people's perspectives, using language that tunes in to their thoughts and feelings. "Your little brother can't stop smiling; he seems to really love playing blocks with you!" Or "The little boy in the story is crying; what do you think he is feeling? What do you think he is going to do next?" Although interacting with your child in this way will by no means ensure his understanding that you need some time to relax (good luck with that one), it will help him learn to better recognize both his own and others' experiences as he grows.

"Why Can't I Handle This?"

Parental Expectations, Baggage, and Emotions

In the last chapter we focused on the different ways in which tantrums are a natural outgrowth of the toddler/preschooler stage of development. That information would be sufficient if your child's meltdowns were occurring in a vacuum. Your little one would begin to have a tantrum, you'd swoop in with your (now) awesome knowledge of child development, say the perfect thing to calm your toddler down, and the two of you would walk gleefully into the sunset holding hands, reveling in the parent–child bliss known only to the characters in Disney movies (except for the ones in which the parents die in the first five minutes, which, in my opinion, is way too many of them, but that's a topic for another book).

Of course, this isn't usually how it goes. Because although (most of the time!) it's your child having the tantrum, the episode is more accurately characterized as an interaction between the two of you. Generally, your child's behavior influences the way you respond, which then influences her behavior, which then influences your response, and so on. This is why, in my practice, I sometimes refer to "tantrum interactions," rather than "tantrums," when working with parents. When we focus too much on what's happening on the child end of things, we miss a crucially important piece of the puzzle: the parent and, more specifically, the way a particular parent experiences and perceives his or her toddler/preschooler. To quote a song from *Free to Be You and Me* (in my opinion, one of the top three children's albums ever made), "Parents are people." And yet, despite this truth, all too often parenting advice—in articles, blog posts, books, or elsewhere—somehow manages to neglect the actual "parent" who's doing all of this parenting. Parents are not abstract beings, generic and interchangeable grown-ups playing a detached and objective role. Rather, they are human beings, each with his or her own unique history, psychological makeup, and emotional life, all of which play an important role in how they experience the aspects of toddlerhood described in the last chapter. And so, to gain a deeper understanding of our child's tantrums, we also have to gain a deeper understanding of ourselves, of what it is that we, as parents, bring to the table.

Let me give you a concrete example. Renee contacted me with concerns about her three-year-old daughter, Olivia. Specifically, Olivia's defiance was "out of control"; it seemed to Renee that every time she asked Olivia to do something, Olivia took pleasure in doing the opposite. Renee would subsequently chastise Olivia, who would then melt down, furious that she was not allowed to do things the way she wanted to. When I asked for examples, Renee rattled off several familiar ones: Olivia wouldn't clean up her toys when she was asked, wouldn't get dressed, wouldn't brush her teeth, wouldn't stop saying "poopie" all the time—the usual. As she spoke, Renee's facial expression became increasingly serious, and the disdain in her voice was nearly tangible. Noticing this, I asked what Renee thought might happen if she approached each of these episodes with a little more playfulness. Renee looked at me, puzzled. I gave a few examples: what if, instead of giving direct commands or corrections, she used humor, games, or contests to bring some levity to moments that would otherwise become fierce power struggles? I watched as Renee's facial expression went from what looked like confusion to disgust and then despair. "Dr. Hershberg," she said quietly, looking down at her hands in her lap, "there is absolutely nothing playful about this."

As I got to know Renee, I learned why Olivia's tantrums were no laughing matter to her. Renee's own mother had struggled with depression during Renee's childhood, and had never been particularly warm, affectionate, or expressive toward her children. Renee couldn't remember an occasion on which her mother had given her a hug or kissed her goodnight. Her mother did, however, show her love through various concrete actions, such as attending Renee's music recitals and driving her long distances to visit her friends (they lived in a rural and somewhat isolated area) Over time, Renee explained, she came to put very little faith in words, to feel that loving someone was about what you *do* for that person, not about what you say or the extent of your emotional warmth and physical affection. When

Olivia defied her, therefore, she took it as a personal rejection, a sign that Olivia's love was lacking. If Olivia loved her, she figured, she would listen to her.

Now, on its face, of course Renee knew this interpretation of Olivia's defiance was somewhat ridiculous. She is a smart, highly educated, and accomplished woman, and on an intellectual level she fully understood that Olivia's defiance was developmentally appropriate rather than personal. And yet she couldn't help feeling deeply wounded each time she battled with her daughter over what were, to her mind, "simple things that Olivia could easily do if she wanted to." Her responses, therefore, came from a place of deep hurt and anger, a place where—not surprisingly—there was clearly no room for any playfulness whatsoever. Furthermore, her hurt and angry responses to Olivia's defiance put an enormous strain on their interactions and relationship, which, of course, only served to make Olivia's behavior worse. Renee came to realize they were stuck in a cycle and that the only way out of it was for her to do some of her own healing so that she could understand, on an *emotional* level, Olivia's behavior for what it was—a developmentally normal (if totally crazy-making) quest for autonomy, *not* a vicious and personal affront.

When I started by providing a strategy Renee could add to her "tantrum prevention repertoire"—in this case, playfulness—I hit a brick wall. She wasn't even able to absorb information about tools, let alone begin to use them, until we cleared up some of her own "stuff" that was getting in the way. And when I say "clear up," please understand that I *don't* mean years of psychotherapy. Which is not to say that wouldn't be helpful, for Renee or anyone else (hey, I'll never discourage anyone from seeking therapy), but just that the simple recognition of how loaded and complicated Olivia's behavior was for her had a powerful effect and freed up space for her to try some new approaches (including, I'm happy to report, playfulness!).

> The "stuff" we all carry into parenting includes our histories, expectations, biases, fears, beliefs—you know, our "stuff."

So how do we begin to look at our roles as parents when it comes to preventing and deescalating our toddlers' tantrums? A lot of it is about the particular tools and approaches we employ, described in Chapters 6–12, and, as you saw in Chapter 3, it's also important to have some foundational knowledge about where young children are in their development. Yet, as you can see from Renee and Olivia, sometimes there are issues pertaining to individual parents that must be recognized or resolved if specific strategies or knowledge about child development are to be of use. In my experience, these issues tend to fall into four different categories: expectations, personal history, current stress level, and emotional reactivity. As you can see, these are awfully broad headings, and a book (or 10!) could be (and has been!) written about each one. What I have found, though—and what I hope you too will discover as you read through the rest of this chapter—is that even a basic understanding of the *general* ways these issues often play out in tantrum interactions can do wonders when it comes to uncovering the *specific* ways this is happening with you and your child.

> To make the best use of knowledge and strategies, get to know yourself: What are your expectations? What did you pick up (and drag along with you) from your childhood? What's your stress level like? How emotionally reactive do you tend to be—or are you at a given moment?

Expectations

There is a great saying that "expectations are resentments under construction," and in my work with parents and young children I've often found this to be the case. When parents hold an expectation of how their child will or "should" act, either in a specific circumstance or more generally, they are essentially laying the groundwork for their own resentment when that expectation is not met. And, frankly, with young children being young children, it's often not met. In turn, once parents feel resentful toward their little ones—that unique blend of bitterness and disdain that feels so incredibly personal—tantrums only get worse. Whether parents voice their resentments explicitly or let them fester silently, toddlers and preschoolers can feel it. Having a sense that your parents resent you (and your inability to meet an expectation you may or may not have known about or have control over in the first place) is a sure path to an emotional meltdown.

The example at the end of Chapter 3, in which your child has a meltdown because you don't rush to his side the second he needs you, is a great example of exactly this. When you are busy and frazzled, it's easy to slip into thinking that your little one can recognize and appreciate this and therefore put his own needs on hold. When he can't—because of the egocentrism and inability to see your perspective that are part and parcel of his stage of development—it's easy to feel resentful. Even if you know your resentment is irrational, the feeling can rear its ugly head. That's the problem with feelings, after all; they just don't abide by logic, no matter how much you wish they would. You may snap at your child for needing you in that moment, knowing, even as the words leave your mouth, that he's not remotely at fault. This, of course, leads him to feel even more upset than he did that you didn't jump at his beck and call in the first place, which then increases your resentment—or, perhaps, at this moment, your guilt kicks in—at which point everyone's emotions are running high and it's all downhill from there. All because of a little expectation that you didn't even know existed!

Expectations can take a lot of different forms. Here are a few that I've encountered (many over and over again) with parents in my practice:

- We expect kids to know things they may not (certain rules, societal norms, etc.).

- We expect sibling number two to behave similarly to the way sibling number one did at the same age.

- We expect our little ones to act like our friends', or siblings', or cousins' little ones do.

- We expect our little ones to be able to keep it together based on our schedule rather than theirs.

- We expect our little ones to act today the way they did yesterday (even when we ourselves aren't always that predictable!).

- We expect our little ones' development to be linear, when, in fact, the path often zigzags (think back to the last chapter and Tommy's fluctuating ability to wait in line for the slide).

- We expect our toddlers and preschoolers to act the way we did when we were little.

- We expect weekends, special occasions (such as holidays), or vacations to be or go a certain way.

- We expect our children's day/week/month (life?) to unfold according to a certain master plan (of which they are unaware).

As you can see, a lot is wrapped up in the expectations we carry with us: social comparisons, the need for control and predictability, attachment to a particular set of outcomes. And the weight of these expectations—that is, the tenacity with which we cling to them—frequently depends so much on the baggage we ourselves carry. Parents who grew up in more chaotic and unpredictable environments, for example, often need, at an almost visceral level, to feel a sense of control and so may adhere quite rigidly to an expectation that their child's development will be linear, say, as a way to feel safe. And yet, as we know from Tommy at the playground, development is not linear, so this expectation is going to get these parents in trouble. Parents from strict families in which they themselves "didn't dare misbehave" (a phrase I hear a lot) may expect their own young children to be similarly self-disciplined, despite having—and *wanting* to have—a more loving and lenient home environment than they had as children. And yet, in loving and lenient environments, toddlers and preschoolers are able to be themselves, which, as we now know, means—among other things— often impulsive and emotional.

The examples are endless. A father who feels insecure about his own rambling career path may, consciously or otherwise, expect his son to be more organized than he's capable of being at age four as a way of shielding him from making the same mistakes Dad did. A tantrum will no doubt erupt when Dad holds him to a standard he can't possibly meet, such as remembering to put his clothes in the hamper every night. A mother unhappy with newfound wrinkles around her eyes may start expecting her daughter to be the most put-together child in the room, as a way of boosting her own struggling self-esteem. (A gender stereotype? Yes. And yet one I see all the time.) When her daughter, as a way of exerting her own budding autonomy, refuses to wear the dress Mom picked out for her, no doubt that tantrum, and the interaction surrounding it, is going to be an intense one.

The "Personal History" section that starts on page 74 takes a deeper dive into some of the most common manifestations of these issues. As with the description of different toddler characteristics in Chapter 3, these topic divisions are meant to be a helpful organizing tool, rather than reflective of how things look in real life, where expectations and personal histories (and numerous other factors) can present as a tangled mess. The expectations we have of our children are no joke, deeply entrenched in our own backgrounds and identities. As such, they are frequently unavoidable, and, frankly, they're not always bad. But a lot of the time, our expectations get in the way. They interfere with our ability to parent effectively, particularly in the case of our children's tantrums. So how do we know if and when this is happening? Easy: when our reactions are harsher than they would be if the expectation were not in place. If you don't *expect* your children to wear particular clothes to parties, or put them in the hamper at the end of the day, you're not quite as frustrated when they don't. If you don't *expect* your son to be on his best behavior at his grandparents' house, you're not quite as upset when he isn't. If you don't *expect* that of course your child will love the beach, you don't feel so irritated when she clearly hates it. If you don't *expect* your child to eat (let alone savor) the delicious dinner you just made him from scratch, you're less likely to snap at him when he takes one bite and declares, "I'm done." If you don't *expect* your child to take only about two weeks to adjust to her new babysitter, you can be more empathic when week three rolls around and she's still having a hard time with her. And when you are not quite as upset or irritated and are less likely to snap, and are more empathic, your little one is less prone to tantrums and more easily soothed overall.

One final note on expectations. As you'll see in Chapter 7, young children actually thrive when the expectations you set for them are clear and conscious, well thought out, and developmentally appropriate. The kind of expectations that hinder rather than help them (and us) give themselves away in their sneakiness. That is, often you don't realize you have them until after the fact. If they made themselves known from the outset, most of us wouldn't have them. No one says, "I expect our upcoming family vacation to go without a hitch, that our toddler will be an absolute gem from start to finish!" And yet parents often have much less tolerance for tantrums on family vacations, starting on day one. Why (aside from the common presence of our own parents or in-laws)? Because, subconsciously, we have the expectation that maybe, just maybe, it'll be an actual vacation this time. Then, when it becomes clear that our kid is still our kid—at home in the living room or on the beach in the tropics—we're disappointed, frustrated, *resentful*. The stakes seem higher, we respond more harshly, and the tantrums get worse. This is even more true when the expectation is a deeper, more entrenched and insidious one.

Unfortunately, there's no magic solution to the issue of sneaky expectations, other than—per usual—your growing awareness of this dynamic at play. As parents, we are never done uncovering our expectations; we need to check them constantly, so that we become more aware when we're clinging to resentments that are under construction. Because resentments under construction over time become fully finished, renovated resentments, then resentment skyscrapers and cathedrals. It's a whole lot harder to tear them down than it is to refrain from building them in the first place.

Personal History

We've already touched on some of the ways that parents' own histories may impact tantrum interactions. In my experience, however, there are three particular aspects of this dynamic that merit a deeper dive, given their relevance to how we respond to and interact around our children's tantrums: the nature of our childhood relationship with our own parents, the extent to and manner in which we were disciplined as children, and the socioeconomic issues with which we grew up (also see the box about the role of culture more generally on page 75).

Our Childhood Relationship with Our Parents

Our relationship with—or *attachment* to—our own parents when we were young, particularly in the first few years, has been shown in study after study to predict the specific ways in which we connect with our own children. (See the box on page 76.)

The case of Renee and Olivia illustrates this idea well. Renee's childhood with a mother who showed her love via actions rather than words led Renee, over the years, to expect and crave the same form of love from others. She (likely both consciously and unconsciously) surrounded herself with adults, including her spouse, who were able to demonstrate their love in this way. When she had Olivia, however, this framework became problematic, especially once Olivia began to test limits and crave autonomy, both of which Renee couldn't help interpreting as personal affronts. When Olivia began to throw normal and developmentally appropriate tantrums, Renee viewed these actions as a *clear and present danger*—that is, evidence that her daughter must not love her. Renee then responded to the tantrums accordingly, which landed mother and daughter in a cycle of anxiety and emotional instability that only contributed to Olivia's having more and more intense tantrums over time.

Another father shared a similar revelation a few sessions into our work. We had been talking about his son's frequent meltdowns and the seemingly disproportionate anxiety he would feel as soon as an episode would begin, anxiety that was paralyzing and prevented him from responding in a productive manner. "Dr. Hershberg," he said to me slowly. "It seems to me that two-year-olds are just like alcoholics. They're just so unpredictable, and that *rage* . . ." His voice trailed off. His own father was a severe alcoholic, and I could almost see the lightbulb go off in his head, comic book

What about Culture?

Obviously, different cultures have different attitudes toward tantrums. In fact, in some cultures there is no such thing as a tantrum. The culture to which you belong—or in which you grew up—may have a great influence on the attitudes you bring to child rearing, and expectations you apply to young children's behavior. The term "culture," is, however, so multifaceted—encapsulating race, ethnicity, nationality, sexuality, religion, language, immigration status, geographic region, military versus civilian, and so forth—that it is impossible to do this factor justice here. You'll see some evidence of its role in the illustrations in this chapter and elsewhere in the book, but for the most part I simply encourage you to think about how tantrums were treated in the environment in which you live or were raised. The point to keep in mind is that if your family and the broader community view tantrums with total tolerance or complete intolerance—or somewhere in between—you probably do too. If the culture in which you grew up framed tantrums in one way and your child's other parent was raised in a different culture with a different attitude about tantrums, there might be a clash. Or you might easily arrive at a comfortable middle ground. Whatever is the case in your home, it's helpful to know the origin of the ideas you bring to the table when it comes to responding to your child's meltdown.

style, as he made this connection. When his son screamed in anger, he was not able to be the calm, centered, present adult he needed to be, because his emotions were actually those of a frightened little boy. His son could sense his father's discomfort, as children are acutely able to do, which then heightened his emotional meltdown, which then increased his father's discomfort. As with Renee and Olivia, there was clearly a cycle in place and one that only this father had the power to interrupt, namely by taking a moment when his son began to melt down to regulate his *own* emotions. He would take a deep breath and internally recite a type of mantra that he came up with for the situation: "The person in front of you right now is your son, not your father. *You* are the father."

Of course, in the interest of full disclosure, when I first suggested using such a mantra, this father laughed. "I think that's the cheesiest thing I've

What Is Attachment Theory and Why Is It So Important?

Put simply, attachment theory, originated by John Bowlby in the 1950s, centers around the idea that, starting at birth, human beings are biologically driven to attach to their primary caregivers. A vast body of research has gone on to link the quality of this attachment to a range of important outcomes for both children and adults, including physical/medical health, psychological well-being, and future peer and romantic relationships. Many experts in the field (developmental, clinical, and public health psychologists, along with pediatricians, psychiatrists, and neuroscientists) posit that a secure attachment to at least one adult in childhood is foundational to healthy development over time. So how do we ensure that our children develop a secure, versus insecure, attachment to us? We acknowledge and meet their needs, both physical and emotional. We do our best to understand who they are and where they're coming from and to meet them where they're at. A hundred percent of the time? Nope. Impossible. We just have to be "good enough," a term coined by Donald Winnicott, a British pediatrician and psychoanalyst, who understood that imperfect parenting, aside from being the only realistic possibility, actually has real benefits for our little ones.

Children who are securely attached are eager and able to explore the world around them, always returning to us, their "secure base," as a source of comfort and support on which they can *predictably rely* again and again. It's not that securely attached children will never have tantrums—in fact, part of feeling safe around their caregivers is knowing on a deep level that they can "let it all hang out," without fear of rejection—but more that, in understanding their tantrums and responding in an emotionally attuned way, parents cement the secure attachment that is so fundamental to their young kids' overall health and well-being.

ever heard," he said. After all, when he had started seeing me a couple of months earlier to add some tools to his parenting toolbox (he and his wife were in the middle of a divorce), reciting a mantra about his own alcoholic father was not exactly what he'd had in mind. That said, I was able to convince him to give it a shot, and it was the first strategy that was actually effective in taming this child's tantrum behaviors. "I told you so!" I joked back when he reported this result. I am not above this.

Here are some other mantras that parents with whom I've worked have adopted to help them remain calm as their children lose it:

- *"She is my child, not my parent; she knows I am a real and important person"* (for the mother who never felt as though her highly traditional parents saw her for her authentic self, and who, therefore, felt particularly triggered when her daughter seemed to be, or was, ignoring her).

- *"Anger is only an emotion; it is not dangerous"* (for the father whose family of origin prided themselves on repressing their feelings, such that anything above a 3 on an emotional intensity scale of 1 to 10 felt foreign and threatening).

- *"I know we will kiss and hug each other goodnight later"* (for the mother who, due to the tenuous connections in her family growing up, felt as though every conflict with her child represented a permanent rupture).

- *"He is not me; I am doing it differently than my parents did"* (for the numerous parents in my practice who project the pain they felt as children onto their own kids, assuming their kids' normal expressions of frustration or sadness must signify deep emotional despair, loneliness, etc.).

One way to "diagnose" that your child's tantrums are somehow triggering your own issues around how you were parented is to ask yourself a simple question, a question I frequently put to my clients as they rant about their frustrations: "How old is the part of you that is having this feeling?" Which is to say, is your reaction coming from your adult self, or does it feel more childlike in nature? If, once you're in a calm and centered

> To reveal the connection between your frustration over a tantrum and your personal history, ask yourself, "How old is the part of me that is having this feeling?"

place, your reaction seems as though it is somehow disproportionate to the circumstances at hand, then the answer is probably the latter. To quote an adage from the 12-step world, "If you're hysterical, it's probably historical."

How We Were Disciplined as Children

Needless to say, there is a great deal of overlap between this aspect of our childhoods and the nature of our childhood relationship with our parents, as described starting on page 74. Nevertheless, it comes up often enough separately and explicitly that it merits its own section, even if only a short one. Essentially, our reactions to our little ones' tantrums are frequently connected directly to the extent to which our own parents set limits on our behavior when we were young children. Sometimes parents had so many limits put on them as children that they allow the pendulum to swing way too far in the other direction. So, for example, Cassie's son, Drew, was having multiple meltdowns per day, primarily due to a lack of structure at home, and the important fact that they worked: a lot of the time, Drew's relentless limit testing resulted in his getting what he wanted. Now, I could have talked to Cassie until I was blue in the face about the importance of setting firmer limits, but until she described a key piece of the puzzle—how she was raised—we weren't going to get anywhere.

> How did your parents discipline you as a child?

It turned out that Cassie's father was a highly religious man, as well as a former military officer. "He controlled every single thing I did," she explained. "I could barely take a breath without asking his permission." Cassie remembered how unpleasant this was for her, how constrained and, at times, shamed she felt, and vowed she was going to do it differently with Drew. Not only did she want to spare Drew the difficult time she'd had, but in this particular case Cassie's father was still alive and an active grandpa, and I had the sense that by treating Drew in the opposite manner to how her father had treated (and, in some ways, continued to treat) her, Cassie was engaging in a type of power play and exacting a certain revenge. The only problem was that Cassie was so clouded by her own "stuff," she couldn't see that Drew, like all children, needed limits, and was, in fact, crying out for them—urgently. But before we could take concrete steps in this regard, imposing structures and routines (and the other approaches outlined in Chapter 7), we needed to talk about how Cassie could do this in a tempered way, without going as far as her own father did and without sacrificing all of the love and warmth in her relationship with Drew (of note, my intention here is not to demonize Cassie's father, who no doubt had his own reasons for becoming the person and parent he became—likely based on his own past experience—but simply to explain how the way in which Cassie experienced and remembered him impacted her parenting of her own child). Once Cassie felt reassured that this was a real possibility, she was able to move forward. She quickly began to respond to Drew's tantrums in much more effective ways, which in turn decreased their frequency and intensity.

Of course, this exact phenomenon can happen in the other direction as well. I've seen many parents who themselves had *no* limits put on their behavior as kids and who, in retrospect, wish their parents had been stricter. They put so many rules and regulations in place that, by the time they've finished listing them all, *I* feel like throwing myself onto the floor in an all-out tantrum. By relying so heavily on the idea that their child "shouldn't be able to get away with what I got away with," they too miss the opportunity to respond to their child's present needs rather than their own unmet past ones.

The important take-home message here is that, in the majority of cases, we don't want to discipline our children in either the exact same *or* exact opposite way that our parents disciplined us. Take the example of a father who was raised in a culture that adhered to the notion that children should be seen and not heard. If this father attempts to replicate this approach fully, he will undoubtedly run into some intense tantrums in his attempts to subdue typical toddler behaviors characterized by autonomy seeking and emotionality (not to mention miss out on some of the delightful expressiveness of young children!). Alternatively, he likely won't land in a better place if he decides that his child needs to be heard *all the time* and consequently makes almost no demands of her, allowing her to run the show. The example may be a bit hyperbolic, but the point is that there is no freedom to be a present, attuned parent in either of these approaches. When we attempt to fully embrace *or* fully reject the way in which we were disciplined as children, our parenting decisions emerge in response to the actions of our family of origin, rather than to those of the family we have created. In doing this, we end up out of sync with our

> Being too rigid about either replicating or rejecting the way we were disciplined takes us out of the present and into the past and weakens our freedom to chart our own course as parents.

little ones, and the relationship suffers. And when the relationship is strained, as you'll see in Chapters 5 and 6, tantrums become more frequent and more intense.

Socioeconomic Issues from Our Childhood

So, this is a complicated one. So complicated, in fact, that I was tempted, more than once, to omit it altogether from this discussion. Whenever issues of wealth or poverty, privilege or the lack thereof rear their heads, it's easy to run in the other direction. And yet, if we do that, we only reinforce their position as the elephant in the room, influencing so much, yet continually unacknowledged. For the parents with whom I have worked—parents of all different socioeconomic backgrounds—this topic often emerges as a critical one, and so it deserves mention. I've given these issues a great deal of thought, both as a child psychologist and as a mother, and have seen their influence manifest in a variety of ways. One difficult interplay occurs when toddlers' normal and developmentally appropriate egocentrism and need for control, described in the last chapter, comes into contact with parents' fear that their children will end up "spoiled" or "entitled."

A personal example this time. My parents came to visit one Sunday afternoon about a year and a half ago, as they often do. Henry ran up to greet my father with unbridled excitement, clutching his new fire engine in both hands and holding it up for him to see. "Grandpa, look! Look!" he gushed, grinning ear to ear. *"Another* toy?" my father responded, ostensibly to him, though clearly (albeit perhaps unconsciously) more for my benefit. (Hi, Dad! You know I think you're amazing in about 25,000 ways, right?) "Yup," Henry responded innocently, unfazed. I, on the other hand, felt my cheeks get warm with shame. My mind began to race, wondering whether I get my kids the things they want too often, about the ratio of *no*s to *yes*es, and jumping ahead to the absolute inevitability of Henry's becoming a horrible adult who has no understanding of the value of money or hard work, unaware that there are children starving in Africa, or that it's important to give back—all because of the new fire engine he got when he was two when it was neither his birthday nor Hanukkah.

Over the next few days, I was firmer than usual when Henry melted down, responding much more rigidly and less empathically than is my typical style. After all, he needed to learn that he couldn't have everything his heart desired, that you don't just get things because you ask for them. Henry's tantrums became more frequent and intense, which only supported my hypothesis that I had been complicit in spoiling Henry, who would now never be able to contribute meaningfully to society. By that Thursday, Henry and I were in a pretty bad rut—it didn't feel good to me, which means he probably felt doubly lousy. I sought some support and soon made the connection between what had happened the prior Sunday with my father and the cycle we were in now. I had been so triggered by my own fears of "spoiling" Henry that my ability to parent in the moment in an attuned, connected way had been compromised. I had never been guilty of parenting in such a way that I gave him everything he wanted, a fact I could see clearly only once the clouds from the prior Sunday had cleared. I had, however, worked hard to be present enough to respond to each request individually and to connect on an emotional level regardless of the content of my response. Henry's tantrums had worsened over the past four days not because he was spoiled but because, overly influenced by my own "stuff," I hadn't been able to connect emotionally and so couldn't calm him down.

The cycle I entered with Henry, stemming from my fear and shame around his becoming spoiled or entitled, is not, of course, unique. Many parents with whom I work—from a range of economic backgrounds themselves—have shared similar concerns and experiences. Of course, I have also worked with clients whose fear is the exact opposite—that their children will feel the same sense of deprivation and, perhaps, consequential shame, that they did when they were younger. I recently met with a couple in which one of the mothers, Janet, was a highly successful investment banker. She had grown up poor on a farm in the rural South and had vivid memories of being made fun of at school for the clothes she wore, which were often ill-fitting, stained, or torn. Now that she had a child of her own, she had vowed that she would never let him want for anything, lest he experience the humiliation she had been made to endure. As a result, when interacting with Janet, her son was able to get everything he asked for, merely by asking. The problem arose when this was not the case with his other mother or with his teachers at preschool. If—and when—these other caregivers attempted to impose limits, he threw a tantrum of the highest magnitude, failing to understand why not everyone let him have everything he wanted the way Janet did. The work with this family was helping Janet see the impact of her own childhood experiences on her parenting decisions and the way in which giving in to her son's every desire was not actually in his best interest. Once she made this connection, she was able to see her son's needs more clearly, and she and her wife were able to get on the same page, consequently decreasing their son's tantrums at home and, ultimately, at school.

Needless to say, these issues—like all the others mentioned thus far in this chapter, frankly—are complicated, defying simple categories or explanations. My hope in at least scratching the surface, however, with a few examples is merely to bring them into your awareness, so that you can start to think about the ways in which your own issues around money, privilege, wealth, and so forth, may be playing out in some way when your child has tantrums. No matter your personal background and current circumstances, there's a real possibility that these issues are one of the many lenses through which you are seeing your little one's "little-ness" and that they are consequently distorting your ability to perceive his or her behavior clearly (a necessary first step to intervening effectively).

Before I move on to the next section of this chapter, I just want to note that this one—the role our own histories play in tantrum interactions—could have included many more subheadings. Food, for example. You know how many toddlers have their worst tantrums at the kitchen table and how many of their parents have issues around food, eating, or body image? A lot. Coincidence? Not so much. Parents who had a hard time making friends as young children will often report that their toddlers' worst tantrums happen in social situations, like the playground or birthday parties. When I probe a bit, sure enough I discover that this is where those parents feel most tense, where the stakes feel highest, and so where they respond most harshly, thus perpetuating, rather than calming, the interaction. I recently met with a mother who told me how self-conscious she was as a child about her lack of athleticism and hand–eye coordination. Guess where her son's most recent meltdown had occurred? You guessed it: on the tennis court, during his very first lesson.

> Where do your sensitivities lie? Is this where a lot of your toddler's tantrums occur?

The point is, we all have parts of our personalities and histories that are sensitive, or easily triggered, and nothing—in both my professional and personal experience—brings them to the surface as quickly and forcefully as our kids' behavior. I have highlighted what I have found to be the most common types of triggers, but please keep in mind that the list is not exhaustive. I just recently met with a mother who was able to stay calm during most of her daughter's tantrums, except when her daughter got so upset that she did "this weird eye thing" (Mom's words), at which point she would fly into a rage. It turned out (which shouldn't surprise you by now) that this mother had struggled with tics as a child and had been teased quite viciously by her elementary school classmates. Once we connected the dots between her rage upon seeing her daughter's eye twitch and her unprocessed emotions about her own childhood experiences, she was able to respond in a different, and calmer, way. Ask yourself if there are similar kinds of connections that you can make. I promise it will be worth your while to spend some time taking inventory of how and where your own stuff might be contributing to your child's meltdowns.

A good place to start would be with the story of your toddler's last tantrum that you wrote after reading Chapter 3, the one that you labeled with the developmentally normal characteristics that your toddler was displaying throughout the interaction. Go back now and note the places where your own issues (around expectations of your child, your relationship with your own parents, the way you were disciplined, socioeconomic factors, etc.) may have been triggered and impacted your responses to your child. What do you notice? Any patterns? Does one issue emerge more than any others?

Depending on your personal style and preference, these issues can be something you commit to thinking about during free moments for the next couple of weeks (maybe while driving or in the shower), or to scheduling some time to talk about with your partner or a close friend. You might journal on these topics and see what comes up. Finally, although it's by no means always necessary, it can certainly be helpful to talk about some of these issues with your own therapist, preferably one who specializes in looking deeply and thoughtfully at parent–child relationships.

So . . . feeling triggered yet? Let's step away from our childhoods, plant our feet firmly in the present moment, and think about something much more concrete: our current stress level. Because, when we're talking about the here and now, few things play a more important role in the interactions we have around our little ones' tantrums.

Current Stress Level

On the surface, this seems like a pretty obvious one, right? Most things become harder when we're stressed, whether it's a conversation with our boss, a disagreement with our spouse, or, frankly, figuring out when to stop at the drugstore to pick up more contact lens solution (I know, I know— order online). When our reserves are low, chores that are typically simple and straightforward become herculean tasks. Our children's behavior is no exception to this rule. When we're running on empty, our attention spans are shorter and our tempers quicker. Our children bear the brunt of this, not only as the frequent direct recipients of our behavior but also because they pick up on our energy and demeanor. And yet I'm constantly surprised by how little attention we pay to our own well-being—our own stress, hunger, and exhaustion levels, for starters—when we think about the role we play in our children's tantrums. We bend over backward to meet our kids' basic needs so as to avoid a tantrum, while not paying nearly enough attention to our own.

Picture the following scenario. You've had a wonderful romantic dinner out with your spouse, gotten several hours of deep and uninterrupted sleep, and are now enjoying a healthy, hearty breakfast. As you get up to put your dish in the sink, you don't notice the Legos in the middle of the kitchen floor and nearly trip over them. Your three-year-old, Sam, is playing in his room. What thoughts go through your head? What do you do? Remember these responses. Now, picture a second scenario. This time, you maybe—*maybe*—got four hours of sleep and are so tired you can barely see straight. In an exhausted frenzy, you shove a Pop-Tart into your mouth and beeline from the pantry to the coffee machine, nearly tripping over the Legos in the middle of the kitchen floor. Again, your three-year-old, Sam, is playing in his room. What thoughts go through your head? What do you do?

When I do this exercise with clients, the gaping difference between the responses elicited by the two scenarios is striking. When parents picture themselves as well rested and well nourished, their thoughts in response to nearly tripping over Legos are so much more forgiving ("Oh, he's only three; of course he doesn't always remember to clean up his toys") and sometimes even complimentary ("Sam is so creative and into building things everywhere he goes"). When asked what they might do in this scenario, they say things like "I would probably just bend down and pick up the Legos myself—it's not that big a deal" or "I'd go to his room and ask him to please come clean up the Legos on the kitchen floor." In contrast, when parents picture themselves as frazzled, tired, stressed—and the kicker, pre-coffee!—their thoughts are much less generous ("That kid is always leaving his toys everywhere I friggin' walk"), and their actions much harsher ("I'd probably yell out that he has to come clean up his Legos *now*").

So, in both scenarios, Sam has committed the same "crime," leaving his Legos on the kitchen floor. And yet, as parents, our reactions are completely different, as is—consequently—the likelihood that Sam will end up throwing a tantrum. Now, I am not here to judge either reaction. I'm simply highlighting that the difference here—between tantrum and no tantrum—is the parent's stress level. Of course we know this intellectually and can pull out our parenting strategies to help (for example, it's preferable to say please and make eye contact when asking your child do something). But if we put a little more effort into being aware of and possibly reducing our stress, we might not have to rely so much on such strategies to begin with. Furthermore—and this is key—most of the time when parents tell me those strategies are not effective, it's because they're used in the midst of peak parental irritation and exhaustion. That is, even if the parent in scenario two *did* walk to Sam's room and request politely that he clean up his toys, it would not be her politeness—as opposed to her impatience and exasperation—that Sam would pick up on. You can't fake generosity of spirit and an ability to empathize with your kid, and both of these come *so* much more easily when you're taking care of yourself.

Unfortunately, given the importance of the concept, the term "self-care" has become overused and even clichéd, reserved for yoga magazines and blogs about meditating. The thing is, though, self-care is not just about taking a bubble bath or getting a massage or manicure, and I actually resent that this has become the implication. Self-care can be as simple as making sure you've had a sandwich, rather than picking up your kid from preschool when you haven't had anything to eat besides a banana

> Generosity and empathy don't feel very authentic when they have to fight their way through irritation and exhaustion.

and a few crackers all day. Or if, for whatever reason, you genuinely have no time or opportunity to have anything other than a banana and crackers all day, at least being *aware* of the impact this will likely have on your interactions with your child on the way home. It's about making sure that somehow, in some way, you don't get too sleep deprived. And about holding on to even just a single interest you had prior to having kids and finding time for it even if only once a month.

If your child's tantrums seem worse, it may be that you're wearing the gray-colored glasses brought about by exhaustion. Or it may be that they actually *are* worse in reality, because you are lacking in the energy and warmth and patience that toddlers and preschoolers demand in such high quantities. Either way, think about the last time you had a good night's sleep, or ate a healthy meal, or did something just for yourself. All three may not be possible right now; you may have a newborn, a demanding new job, or a new aversion to vegetables. But it's important to prioritize doing something to take care of you. Your kids will thank you.

One of the reasons (although not the only one) that our sleep is so important with regard to how we interact with our little ones around tantrums is the relationship between sleep deprivation and increased emotional reactivity. Specifically, research shows that when we haven't slept enough, our emotional reactions become longer, more frequent, and more intense than they would be otherwise—findings that won't surprise any of you, I'd imagine. Of course, there are plenty of other reasons that people are more or less emotionally reactive as well, but, regardless of how we get there, I have seen time and time again that the level of parents' emotional reactivity influences how they interact with their toddlers around tantrums, which, in turn—as usual—affects the tantrums themselves.

Emotional Reactivity

A couple of months ago I was sitting in my office with new clients, Greg and Sandra, conducting an intake session about the difficulties they were having with their daughter's behavior. About 25 minutes into the session, Greg's phone vibrated, and he apologized to me before taking it out of his pocket. Upon looking at the screen, he suddenly shouted, "Oh, F*%K!" I jumped in my chair, startled by the abruptness and volume (let alone profanity) of his exclamation. Of course, I immediately asked if everything was OK. "Yeah, I just have to reschedule a meeting," he responded bitterly, his facial expression having shifted to a noticeably more negative demeanor. "He always gets like this," Sandra quickly followed up.

You likely have many of the same initial questions I did in that moment. Was this a particularly important meeting? Were the stakes unusually high? Had Greg put in a great deal of effort scheduling it in the first place? Would rescheduling be particularly labor intensive for some reason or other? The answer, over and over again, was no. Rather, what came out was that Greg was just a very emotionally reactive person. He had big reactions to things—positive and negative—and, once he was triggered in a particular direction, it took him a while to come back to center. Nothing about Greg was, to use more colloquial descriptions, "laid back" or "even keel." And, although this quality ebbed and flowed to a degree, it was, for the most part, a rather stable part of who he was and how he both experienced and interacted with the world. His daughter's tantrums, of course, were no exception.

There are a variety of reasons that, at any given moment in time, some people are more emotionally reactive than others, not only when it comes to their current mood or *state* (which, as discussed, may depend on stress, exhaustion, triggers pertaining to childhood history), but also with regard to their general temperament and personality (that is, a more stable *trait*). For the purposes of this discussion, however, the *why*s aren't necessarily that important. What *is* critical, however (and you're probably sensing a trend here), is to develop some level of insight about where you, as a person, fall on this continuum. Forgetting about parenting for a moment, think about something much more basic: driving. What are you like when someone cuts you off during a typical, everyday (read: not emergency-related) drive? Are you pretty easy-breezy about it, effortlessly letting it roll off your back? Or does your whole body clench up with rage, leaving you still ruminating about *just how wronged you were* 30 minutes later? Certainly, your answer may be "it depends," but a lot of the time people see themselves as, at least on a typical day, fitting more generally into one category or the other. Greg certainly did, once we had the conversation, which is also (not coincidentally, of course) when he was able to have a clearer sense of the role he played in exacerbating his daughter's emotional meltdowns.

If a parent is someone who is quick to anger, then, as you can imagine, a child's tantrum is a clear and obvious impetus. After all, if Greg's rage kicked in when he was faced with a smartphone notification about a meeting, what must he have been like when confronted by his daughter's defiance or rigidity? A powder keg, that's what. Every time his daughter had a meltdown, Greg would fly off the handle in a way that only made the tantrum worse. And so, in this case, Greg needed to do some real work around learning how to regulate his own emotional reactions before he could effectively use some of the more concrete strategies and approaches outlined later in this book. He learned certain mindfulness strategies, for example, that enabled him to tune into bodily cues that he was about to lose his temper (such as his increased heartbeat and the tightness in his chest) and then various relaxation practices (breathing, for example) he could use to calm himself down. Only then would he interact with his daughter around her tantrum.

With time, this process got faster and more automatic for him. In the interim, though, he narrated his actions out loud, thereby modeling an incredibly important set of skills for his daughter. "OK," he would say, "my chest just got tight, which means I am feeling really frustrated and am probably going to yell soon. *Feeling* frustrated is OK, but the *behavior* of yelling at you isn't. I don't want to do that. Instead, I am going to take three deep breaths." At first, Greg was embarrassed for his daughter to see him undergoing this learning process, but we soon reframed this as a tremendous gift, something that became clear the first time he saw his daughter join him in the practices—counting and breathing along with him. Calming our bodies and our minds takes effort and practice, and it turned out that Greg could be a real teacher for his daughter in this extraordinarily important area.

> Your own emotional reactivity offers you an opportunity to validate your preschooler's feelings while modeling skills for emotional regulation.

As you think about the role you play in responding to your child's tantrums, it bears reiterating that—much like the toddler and preschooler characteristics outlined in the last chapter—these areas can (and often do) overlap and intersect. You may be losing your temper with your son of late due to some combination of all of the above: you're a pretty emotionally reactive person to begin with, he's more difficult than his older sister was, his unpredictability reminds you of the crazy moods your own father had when you were little, you're worried about letting him get away with too much, you fear he's getting "spoiled," you've barely slept in a week, and you've been subsisting on a diet of caffeine, wine, and your children's leftovers. The point of looking at each of these areas separately is not to create a contrived scenario in which human reactions are oversimplified, but, rather, to help you understand some of the variables that may be at play during the worst interactions you have with your little one. It has been my experience time and time again that only by diving into some of this—going a bit deeper than you might have imagined—will you be able to effectively implement the actual concrete strategies for preventing and managing tantrums that are put forward in the chapters to come.

Q "I get that it's important to recognize my own personal triggers, but sometimes I feel like anyone would be triggered in my situation. For example, when my daughter says 'I hate you' during a tantrum, aren't I right to be triggered by that? I feel so hurt and angry, but who wouldn't?"

A This is a question I hear a lot. A child says "I hate you," or "I like Mom better than you," or "I wish you weren't my mom," in the lead-up to or during a tantrum, and a parent describes feeling wounded and reacting in a combination of hurt and fury. And how can we not?

The response is completely natural. And yet, when young children say these things, they are expressing their anger and frustration in what is, for the most part, a developmentally appropriate way. And I believe (others may, of course, disagree) that the expression of emotion is something to be encouraged, rather than suppressed. After all, I want Henry and Zeke, when they're teenagers, to *tell* me when they're angry at me about something and for us to be able to talk it out, rather than for them to act out behind my back. Unfortunately, though, in these moments, parents often end up responding in a way that makes the situation worse, not better. For example:

- "You are not allowed to speak to me that way, young man!" Sounds powerful, sure, but having a conversation about manners when everyone's emotions are running high is never an effective strategy. It's almost a guarantee that this kind of response will escalate rather than defuse the situation.

- "That hurts my feelings." On the one hand, this is true, sure. On the other, it gives our children's feelings an awful lot of power, implying they are somehow dangerous. Your children are not responsible for protecting your feelings; this is an unhealthy role reversal.

- "No you don't." This is invalidating. Your child *does* feel that way—hating you, preferring Mom, whatever—in that moment, and remember, as seen in Chapter 3, that moment is all that exists to him!

- "We only use kind words in our home." This is aspirational, but not the way humans work. It's important to have ways of expressing less-than-kind feelings, and, when you're a toddler or preschooler, one way to do this is by using less-than-kind words. If adults in the home model better skills for coping with conflict or difficult feelings, children ultimately learn them too. Not by age five, though. Even thirty-five is a stretch for some. ☺

- "Hate is a bad word" or "We don't believe in hate." I have never understood this, to be honest. Hate exists. It's on the continuum of emotion—the opposite of love, a more extreme version of dislike. In my opinion, it's OK to feel hate, primarily because I don't think we have control over this, the same way we don't have control over a lot of the emotions we experience. How is saying we "don't believe in hate" any different from saying we "don't believe in love"? And yet I hear the former all the time. What's not to believe in? It exists. It's real. Let's accept and work with it. (Stepping off soapbox now.)

- "Well, I like Mom better than *you!*" Only including this because a father once confessed—embarrassed and ashamed—that he said this to his daughter. *We. Are. All. Human.* He asked me if their relationship would ever recover. It did. They are really close.

So how do we respond in these trying moments? As parents, it's up to us to begin to teach our young children emotion words—mad, angry, frustrated—as well as to help them label and make sense of their emotional experiences so that slowly they can learn to do so themselves (more on this in Chapter 8). I generally recommend taking a deep breath and saying something like:

- "I see that you're so mad at me right now. You seem really frustrated that I asked you to clean up when you want to keep playing. You love playing with your cars *so* much."
- "You really thought you were going to be able to watch another show, and I said no. That stinks, and so you feel really disappointed and angry, right?"

By responding in this way, you're helping your child create a narrative around, and therefore understand and accept, her emotional experience. You're not allowing your own hurt or anger to be dominant or to dictate your response in a counterproductive way. You can continue to set the limit that prompted your child's reaction, and perhaps later, when cooler minds prevail, you can have a repair in which you talk about the fact that we can love a person and still feel angry at him or her at the same time. More on all this good stuff in the chapters to come!

5

"Maybe If Things Were Just a Bit Less Crazy on the Home Front..."

Family Dynamics and the Foundation for Reducing Tantrums

At this point it should be obvious that tantrums don't emerge out of nowhere but rather as interactions between parents and children. There's more, however: the interactions that parents and toddlers or preschoolers have during the course of a tantrum don't occur in a vacuum either. Real life is complicated. You may be cruising along just fine with your toddler, handling tantrums like a champ with your newfound knowledge of brain development and Zen mastery over your own triggers, but then—just when you're starting to get cocky—something happens, and it feels like you're right back where you started. Your child's tantrums once again become more frequent and intense, and you're losing your temper left and right. It feels like there's been a major setback, and you don't really understand why. What's happening?

Until this point, we've thought about the interactions between toddlers and parents as a sort of dance that occurs throughout the day. For the dance to proceed the way we want it to—as smoothly and gracefully as possible, with tantrums that are as few and far between, minor, and short-lived as possible—you need to have a good understanding of what each participant (child and parent) contributes along the way. For example, as a mother, I need to know that my three-year-old Henry's developmental stage is characterized by (among other things) a craving for autonomy and high emotionality. I also need to be aware of my own "stuff," such as the expectations I put on him without always realizing it and the way in which

91

some of my parenting choices are disproportionately influenced by certain aspects of my own childhood. A lot of the time, if I keep these two knowledge bases in mind, I can predict the dance between Henry and me, as well as control (at least to an extent) its outcome. Sometimes, however, while always important, this step alone is insufficient, and we need to go one step further and look at the chemistry between the two dancers. When are their dance styles complementary, and when do they seem to be missing each other somehow? In the child development world, this idea is known as *goodness of fit*.

The Parent–Child Dance: Goodness of Fit

"Goodness of fit" is a term that can apply to an individual parent–child dyad as well as a larger family system. The term emerged from research done in the 1970s on the importance of an infant's temperament—the way the baby responds to the surrounding environment, on both a physiological and an emotional level. Children are born with a specific way, or style, in which they approach the world, including, for example, their emotional intensity, frustration tolerance, reaction to new people or situations, and general activity level. When parents say their child "came out of the womb" a certain way—loving loud music, very cautious around new people, or with a ton of excess energy—it's a pretty sure bet they're talking about a facet of temperament. Think back to our discussion of emotional reactivity in Chapter 4, to Greg, whose sudden, loud, and profane exclamation upon learning his meeting was canceled caught me off guard, at which point his wife noted that this reaction was actually typical for him. Based on my observations, and later affirmed by his account, Greg was high on *intensity,* one of the nine temperament traits that have been described by researchers (see the box on page 93 and the Resources for leads to more information).

Goodness of fit, then, refers to the extent to which there is congruence between the temperament with which a child is born and the environment the baby is born into. Within the parenting context, a "good fit" describes the interaction between temperament and parenting style in particular; parents see, understand, and accept their child's intrinsic nature and then parent accordingly. A "poor fit" occurs when, conversely, parents parent from a place of misunderstanding, lack of acceptance, or disrespect for a child's natural temperament. A large body of research suggests that a "good fit" is correlated with a range of positive outcomes for kids, from healthy

How Do We Define Temperament?

Scientists have identified nine specific traits that combine to form an individual's temperament. Where do you think you and your child(ren) fall—high or low—on the continuum of each of these traits?

- Intensity
- Activity level
- Distractibility
- Regularity
- Sensitivity
- Approach/withdrawal
- Adaptability
- Persistence
- Mood

self-esteem to emotion regulation skills, flexibility, and a sense of belonging.

You have probably already guessed where this is going, but tantrums are likely going to be more frequent and more intense in families where there is a poor fit between a child's temperament and a mother's or father's parenting style, and, more specifically, in settings or situations in which this incongruence is particularly apparent. Let me give you an example. When Paulette first came to see me about her daughter Tess's tantrums, she described them as being primarily problematic during social situations, such as at the playground or birthday parties. When in these situations, Tess frequently clung to Paulette's leg, and when Paulette urged her to go and play with her friends, Tess would suddenly, and seemingly without warning, "go from zero to sixty," melting down wholly and completely. As I learned more about both Paulette and Tess, I realized there was an issue of "poor fit" at play. Specifically, Tess was a child who was slow to warm up (a term pertaining to the approach/withdrawal temperament trait, used to describe a set of kids who tend to approach the world somewhat cautiously); she was guarded in new situations, even when she knew everyone present. Paulette was on the other side of the approach/withdrawal continuum; she was a true extrovert and always had been. She loved meeting new people (the more the merrier) and had a really difficult time putting herself in the shoes of someone who felt otherwise, particularly her own child. Rather than accept Tess for who she was in this regard, Paulette was in the habit of pushing her too hard too quickly, leading Tess to feel compounded discomfort; not only was she nervous about the situation at hand, but she also could feel, almost tangibly, just how much her mother didn't "get" her, and at times even disapproved of her.

My work with Paulette focused on helping her both to recognize and to accept her daughter's temperament, including her own feelings and reactions. Because, although no temperament is inherently better or worse than any other, there are undoubtedly certain characteristics that some people and/or cultures value more or less, and it's important to acknowledge rather than deny this truth. Not only was Paulette herself an extrovert, but she was raising her child in a Western culture, which—while this is a generalization—tends to place a high premium on extroversion, that is, on being outgoing, confident, vocal, and self-assured. I see this in my practice when parents feel elated to learn, at their parent–teacher conference, that their preschooler is a "natural leader" in the classroom, as contrasted with the disappointment parents report upon hearing their little one is often shy, or private. I would argue—fervently and passionately—that our world needs both, and yet the difference in parent reactions is striking. It is not a surprise then, that for reasons influenced by both her personal experiences and the surrounding culture, Paulette worried, for example, that her daughter's being slow to warm up in social situations would negatively impact her future success in the school and professional realms.

> Could your child's tantrums be related to the child's being on the opposite end of the continuum for a temperament trait that you value very highly?

During our subsequent work together, we talked about the fact that, although we are each indeed born with a certain temperament, these traits alone do not determine our personalities, which are also vastly influenced by the environment in which we're raised and, in particular, interactions with our primary caregivers. The best analogy I've heard to illustrate this, although certainly an oversimplification, is that of a cake. A child is born as batter, the ingredients of which are fixed; whether or not he or she "rises" to become a cake depends on the cake pan, the oven temperature, how closely the mixing and baking of the batter is monitored, and so on. To take the analogy one step further,

Paulette's attempts to get Tess to be more social at parties were akin to her attempting to turn the batter for a soufflé into brownies made from a mix. They were not acknowledging the essence of who Tess was and were not made delicately enough to enable Tess to flourish. (Here, it is important to note that I myself am not a baker, although even I can pull off brownies from a mix, which is why I use that example.)

It can be easier for us to parent a child whose essence (temperament, batter, whatever) resembles our own; we know, on a much more innate level, what to do. When our child's temperament differs from our own, so there's the potential for a poor fit, it is not that all hope is lost but that we need to learn how to help our child thrive the way *she* is going to thrive, not the way *we* did per se. In Paulette's case, she needed to recognize and accept that Tess was never going to be the life of the party; it just wasn't who she was born to be. And to the extent that she had always dreamed her daughter would take after her in this way, she needed to experience the emotions that came with letting go of that fantasy. And then she needed to learn how to help Tess, as Tess, come out of her shell, to parent in a more gentle and attuned manner, one that signaled her support, rather than disapproval, of the way in which Tess navigated her world.

For example, instead of making it seem as though entering a birthday party was an objectively super-fun activity, Paulette needed to acknowledge that it could, in fact, feel scary. Rather than pry Tess's fingers from her leg immediately and abruptly, she needed to allow Tess to move slowly, first allowing her to cling to her leg, then holding her hand instead, then standing by her side, and only then, perhaps, encouraging her to take a few steps by herself toward the action of the party *all while making it clear she was on her team.* That piece is key. Paulette learned to put her own judgment aside and to see the world through Tess's eyes. She learned to help Tess master "brave skills," instead of invalidating her worries. She learned to communicate an unconditional enjoyment of being with Tess during social situations, no matter how Tess acted, and to "bookend" them with connectedness and affection. Within a few months, despite their ongoing temperamental differences, the relationship between Tess and Paulette had greatly improved, and Tess's tantrums decreased notably in both frequency and intensity.

> Temperament differences do not have to result in a poor fit.

Other common temperament/personality "mismatches" I've encountered in my practice include:

- The rough-and-tumble son with the shy, artsy dad
- The pretty-in-pink princessy daughter with the couldn't-care-less-about-fashion mom
- The love-to-be-outdoors mom with the love-to-be-indoors son
- The love-to-be-indoors dad with the love-to-be-outdoors daughter
- The always-on-the-go daughter with the sit-on-the-couch-and-read mom
- The shoot-'em-up son with the on-the-board-of-Everytown-for-Gun-Safety mom
- The foodie dad with the all-chicken-nuggets-all-the-time son
- The deep-and-intense-feelings daughter with the things-roll-off-my-back, easy-breezy dad
- The it's-not-fun-unless-it's-dirty son with the germ-phobic mom

Sometimes It's Just a Phase . . . or Just the Time or Place

Needless to say, not all of the examples in the list above pertain to temperament or even general personality. Many—get ready to breathe a sigh of relief!—reflect mere passing phases. A lot of four-year-old girls enjoy dressing up as princesses for a period of time and then move on to other activities as they grow up. Similarly, young kids often experiment with "guns" (store-bought toys or, often to parents' dismay, a stray branch lying on the ground) when they are figuring out the different roles one can play in the world, the concepts of "good guys" and "bad guys," superheroes and villains, real and pretend. This is a normal part of development, and frequently, as children get older, their interest in weapons and shooting and killing goes by the wayside. Still, each of these examples taps into how parents' ways of being in the world—or tastes, interests, or preferences—may diverge significantly from those of their child.

Sometimes these incongruences pop up only at certain times (such as during meals or playground games), and in other situations they're more pervasive, coloring the whole parent–child relationship. Either way, one of the most important interventions I do with these families is to help parents see and appreciate their children for who they are at a given moment in time and to create opportunities that deepen their connection rather than emphasize their differences. If two dancers aren't feeling the chemistry, after all, sometimes it's just about changing the lighting or the music, right?

So now, let's say we've got our young child and our parent dancing well together, in a good rhythm, able to prevent (and deescalate, as necessary) tantrums gracefully and skillfully. Until—dum-DUM (that's my feeble attempt to capture the opening music of *Law and Order* in writing)—a third person wants to join the dance! And everyone knows that dancing in a group of three—or four, or five—is a lot more complicated. It's one thing to figure out the box step with your partner, but a whole other task when we're talking the Electric Slide, the hora, or insert-your-cheesy-wedding-group-dance-of-choice-here!

Line or Group Dancing: The Role of Families

A lot of the time, families are not comprised of only a single parent and single toddler. Often, there are two parents, siblings, stepparents, grandparents, nannies . . . the list of possible players goes on. And because of that, it's impossible to illustrate the impact of every possible family permutation on tantrums. If your quest, however, is to understand what's behind your toddler's tantrums, then you'd be remiss in neglecting to take into consideration larger family dynamics.

Siblings

I recently did an observation of a family with twin three-year-old boys, Andy and Ilan, to help their parents understand why it was that Ilan was having so many more tantrums than Andy at home (he was great at school). I watched as their father, who had just gotten home from work, sat down to do a puzzle with the boys before dinner. After a few minutes, Ilan seemingly got bored with the activity and walked over to the toy area, ostensibly to find something else to do. Within moments he was stamping on the floor, declaring angrily, "I *hate* these toys! I don't want to play with *anything*!" The twins' father immediately ceased doing the puzzle with Andy to attend to Ilan's outburst, at first just verbally from where he was and then physically as well, joining Ilan in the toy area to chastise him for his tone of voice. Andy continued working on the puzzle by himself.

I have seen this type of interaction over and over again. A parent is playing nicely with one sibling, at which point the other sibling begins to melt down about something or other. The parent will stop playing, quickly attending to the sibling causing the commotion to stave off any further upset. Sometimes, of course, this is both necessary and warranted, especially if there's the chance that the child having a hard time is in genuine distress. In other cases, however, this type of interaction signifies a larger, more problematic pattern, in which children learn that the way to get their parents' attention most easily and efficiently is through tantrum behaviors. Over time, this creates sibling "roles," whereby one child becomes known as the "more difficult" one, often receiving a disproportionate amount of parental focus. And, as we know from Chapter 2, even if this focus comes in the form of scolding or exasperation, it can be reinforcing to a child, thus putting into place a cycle that ultimately doesn't serve anyone involved. (Sibling relationships, of course, are much more complicated than I can address here, and I've given some good resources for more information at the back of the book.)

Two-Parent Families

To understand Ilan's tantrums, it was imperative to look at his behavior within the family context, which is very frequently the case in families with more than one child. This scenario, however, in which sibling roles become dominant in explaining the emergence of tantrums, is merely one of countless family dynamics that can play an important role. Another key variable to explore, and that frequently comes up in my practice, is the nature of the adult partnership that exists within two-parent families. Although parents can be, and hopefully are, valuable sources of support to each other, there is also the potential for one's partner to become one's adversary, particularly around parenting issues. Even in generally healthy partnerships, parents may come from opposite places with regard to parenting philosophies or preferred child-rearing approaches, which can create a great deal of tension. And when there is tension between parents, particularly (although not exclusively) around issues pertaining to parenting, you can count on the fact that kids will pick up on it and that their behavior— in this case tantrums—will be impacted significantly.

Let's take the example of two fathers, Michael and Geoffrey, whom I currently see in my practice. Both adore their two-year-old daughter, Meena, but they have very different ideas about parenting. Michael, who was raised by a single mother in a not particularly safe part of Baltimore, believes in strict discipline and that children do best when they feel "a little bit afraid" of their parents. Geoffrey, who grew up in a two-parent family in a wealthy suburb of Los Angeles, cannot comprehend Michael's perspective and wants only to comfort and nurture their daughter when Michael imposes firm limits. Two parents, both with the best of intentions, each coming to the parenting table with his own upbringing, culture, and set of experiences. They reached out to me because Meena had begun to play them off against one another, highly aware—even at age two—that Michael was the "bad cop" and Geoffrey was the "good cop." Her tantrums, which occurred when she didn't get something she wanted, had become very difficult to handle, and her parents couldn't agree on the best way to manage them.

Michael and Geoffrey frequently argued overtly during Meena's tantrums. "Why can't she have just one more cookie?" Geoffrey would ask angrily. "It's not like we're giving her a whole cake!" "Because we already told her no and she needs to know we mean it!" Michael would retort. And this would continue, all within earshot of Meena. As the conflict between Michael and Geoffrey heightened, her tantrum would worsen, likely for two main reasons. First, she could perceive her parents' anger at each other, as well as the fact that her behavior was at the source. Feeling as though one's emotions and related behavior are somehow "too much" for one's parent(s) can be extremely anxiety provoking for children, which only increases their distress and tantrum behavior. Second, because Meena was aware of the good cop/bad cop dynamic, she had also learned that, at least some of the time, if she persisted in her tantrum, she would ultimately get what she wanted, in this case another cookie.

> Is the fit between your parenting style and the other parent's style fueling tantrums?

My work with Michael and Geoffrey was, therefore, twofold, as is often the case when I meet with parents who harbor such different parenting philosophies. The first goal was to insist (yes, in cases like this I can be *that* directive!) that they curtail the arguing in front of their daughter. It was certainly OK for Meena to see her parents disagree at times, of course, but not for her to be exposed to what had become nasty disagreements specifically about how to handle her behavior. What Meena needed to feel was that the grown-ups were in control and were presenting a united front. The second goal was to work with Michael and Geoffrey on finding common ground between their two parenting styles, so that each could be part good cop and part bad cop and Meena could experience both as sources of nurturing and structure. Sure enough, once these two goals were achieved— although goals are always, obviously, works in progress to some extent— Meena's tantrums became fewer and farther between.

Once again, the point is not that every two-parent family mirrors Michael and Geoffrey, but merely that the tantrum dance is not limited to an individual toddler and individual parent and that you frequently have to look at these larger family variables to arrive at the source of tantrums. (As with siblings, the impact of the relationship between parents on their kids is too complicated to address in full here; see the Resources for sources of more information.) Ask yourself: Who else has joined in to dance with you and your toddler at the most problematic times? Because when you start to see all of the dancers and their respective moves clearly you really start to see the factors that likely rest at the heart of your child's tantrums. That is, of course, until the music changes or the ground starts to shift. Seriously.

 "I'm the good cop, and my partner is the bad cop. Is that bad? It works for our family."

 Whenever people tell me that something is working for their family, so long as no one is in abject emotional or physical danger, I take a step back. After all, families vary widely, and it's not my role (or style, frankly) to judge what works or doesn't work for different people in different circumstances. You do you, as they say. That said, people generally come to me precisely because something *isn't* working, which is also, I presume, why many of you chose to read this book. It's my job to connect the dots, so if your child is having very difficult tantrums, and you believe it has nothing to do with the good cop/bad cop system of discipline you're using—intentionally or because you just kind of fell into it based on who felt comfortable in what role—one of the things I do is highlight the ways in which there could very well be a connection. What good cop/bad cop does, in effect, is assign one parent to "Love" and the other to "Limits." That doesn't mean that both parents don't offer some degree of both, but when things get stressful—for example, in the lead-up to or during a tantrum—the roles become delineated. One could argue, therefore, that in a two-parent family, the child is still getting both "L words," and so what's the problem? From the perspective of the child, put most simply, the problem is the inconsistency. When the two grown-ups in the home perceive and/or handle children's expressions of emotion (the most basic definition of tantrums) and behavior differently, it can be quite confusing and destabilizing. Instead of feeling secure across the board, experiencing their world as predictable and safe (feelings they need to have to explore, learn, grow, and succeed), young children learn that the rules aren't dependable, that it's unclear who's in charge, and that the emotional climate of the home is variable. Children often internalize these feelings, which are stressful for developing brains and can result in later emotional or behavioral issues. In addition to these issues, I've often seen good cop/bad cop approaches divide families in unhealthy ways and cause resentment to fester between parents over time, even if not at first.

When I work with families in which one parent gravitates toward the role of taskmaster or disciplinarian, and the other to nurturer or the "fun one," I frequently ask parents to play around with dividing these roles more evenly. I ask the taskmaster to refrain from making a single demand for a whole Sunday afternoon, for example, focusing only on play and humor. Or I ask the "fun one" to be responsible for taking the kids through the morning or evening routine the next day. Sometimes parents experience anxiety merely speaking about these role shifts and express resistance. These conversations often become rich sources of information about couple and family dynamics and about parents' individual backgrounds and triggers. And, as you've heard me say before (and will hear me say again), building awareness around these various and complex issues is key to the prevention and deescalation of tantrums.

Q "Is it ever OK for parents to fight in front of their children?"

A Yes, although I prefer to use the word "argue" or even the phrase "show conflict." The important thing to know here is that researchers have distinguished between different types of parental conflict. When parents use hostile and destructive tactics with each other during conflicts, the risks for children can be significant, including a range of emotional, behavioral, and health problems. These tactics include physical and verbal aggression, "silent tactics" (such as avoidance or withdrawing), and capitulation. Avoiding conflict altogether, however, is not the solution, in part because it's impossible. There's no way that two adults who live together, let alone raise children and a family together, can relate in authentic, connected ways without having disagreements and some conflict. The answer, it turns out, is to model healthy ways of coping with conflict, including negotiation and compromise, as well as demonstration of support and the expression of positive emotions. Not only is witnessing this type of constructive conflict not harmful for kids, but it's actually linked to some positive outcomes, including increased emotional security, social skills, and self-esteem. All couples have conflict; it's whether it's constructive or destructive that matters when it comes to children.

If you are experiencing destructive conflict in your partnership, I recommend seeking professional help in the form of a couples thera-pist (see the Resources, "Getting Professional Help" section, for how to find someone). If your conflict is constructive, I highly recommend a strategy I learned about in an article by Diana Divecha, one that the author used in her own family. When you are arguing with your part-ner and your toddler or preschooler shows or voices some concern, you can reassure him by holding your fingers an inch apart: "This is how big the fight is." Then throw your arms open wide: "But *this*? This is how big the love is."

What Happened to the Music?: The By-the-Way Factor

With an understanding of how other parties factor into the potential-tantrum dance, you're even closer to having a "formula" for keeping a lid on toddler meltdowns. But wait. What about the music? And the dance floor? We can only understand and direct the dance of tantrum interac-tions *if*—and this is a really big if—the ground is stable and the rhythm is steady. When we're talking about tantrums, the ground and the music are the surrounding environment, the context in which the tantrum occurs. Because no matter how well you come to know your toddler's dance moves, as well as perfect your own and observe those of the others around you, there is a never-ending list of environmental factors you can't control that may well knock you off your feet.

I call this list the "by-the-way factors." Why? Because of the number of voice mails and emails I receive in which these environmental factors are referenced as an afterthought, as if they could not possibly explain the uptick in tantrums but are *perhaps* worth mentioning just in case. Here's a sampling of the type of information that, over the years, parents have casu-ally tacked on to the end of an expression of concern about their toddler's tantrums:

- "Oh, and by the way, I should also mention that I'm 35 weeks pregnant with our second child."
- "I doubt this has anything to do with it, but my husband just lost his job, and so things have been pretty tense around the house."
- "Also, just as an aside, we got two new puppies about a week ago."
- "I almost forgot to mention it, but my grandfather actually moved in with us last month; yeah, he was in Texas and his house got flooded in the hurricane there."
- "Oh, and also she just had her tonsils out."
- "I'm sure it's not important, but our social calendar has been insane; my wife and I have been out almost every night this past week."
- "I meant to ask you: can in-laws cause tantrums? Because everything I just described happened when we were at my husband's parents' last weekend, just in case that's important."
- "I had a miscarriage right around the time he started acting out at bedtime, but he didn't know, so I can't imagine it's related."
- "By the way, we're moving next week, so all our stuff is in boxes."
- "I should also just mention that our nanny quit totally unexpectedly about a month ago—she just never showed up one morning."
- "I'm sorry—can you repeat that? Our smoke alarm is going off again. It's been doing that sporadically every hour or so for the past couple of days. Wait, could that have anything to do with this?"

In therapy parlance, remarks like these are frequently referred to as "doorknob comments" or "doorknob revelations." Why? Because therapy clients often leave the most important piece of information until the very end of the session, when they're literally walking out of the room, and so have their hand on the doorknob. Same too with these "by-the-way factors." More often than not, despite the nonchalant, easy-breezy tone with which they're introduced, these pieces of information have *everything* to do with why children's tantrums have become more frequent or intense. After all, remember that tantrums are behavioral manifestations of overwhelming emotions, and nearly everything referenced in the list above could very well lead a two- or three-year-old to experience really big and overpowering feelings.

Needless to say, the list above represents merely a sampling of possible issues or events that can come up and lead to an increase or worsening in a toddler's or preschooler's tantrums. My point was not to be comprehensive (in this case, a not only laborious but also impossible task given the infinite possibilities), but rather to point out the importance of doing your detective work. If your little one's tantrums seem to be getting inexplicably worse, and you've already looked at the various possible contributors we've discussed thus far, it's time to look carefully at the outside context, at what's going on in your home, family, neighborhood, or community that may be having a direct or indirect impact on the interactions around tantrums, or the dance you're in. There just might be a variable you've been tossing off in your mind as no big deal that's actually key to understanding your child's tantrums of late.

 "Could my son's tantrums really have gotten worse because I had a miscarriage? How is this possible? I was barely even pregnant, and we never even told him!"

 This particular query pertains to a miscarriage, but I've heard the same type of question with regard to a range of other difficult/stressful events and circumstances (see the question about a grandmother's illness on page 225 in Chapter 12). The question, more generally, is how on earth young children's behavior—in this case, tantrums—can be impacted by things about which they are never told and clearly don't know. Six words: *your child is on to you.* Toddlers and preschoolers are sponges. Their brains are constantly looking for new information, learning, exploring, taking in their environments. Their eyes and ears and minds and hearts are always working, picking up cues, energy, changes in facial expressions, tones of voice around them. All of which is to say that if something occurs in your family that impacts the general atmosphere—mood, energy, routine, emotional climate—your young children are going to know it, even if their knowledge is neither concrete nor conscious. And when they pick up on a change they don't understand, or that doesn't feel good in some way, it can be emotionally overwhelming. Where there's emotional overwhelm, an increase in tantrum frequency and severity is often not far behind.

So what do we do? Clearly, we're not going to tell our two-and-a-half-year-old that Mommy was pregnant for five weeks but that the pregnancy was not a healthy one and so it didn't take. What we can do, however, is acknowledge to our children that we are feeling sad because of something that happened that had nothing to do with them. We can add that being sad sometimes is OK and that we are talking to other grown-ups about it to feel better. This way, our child is reassured that she is not crazy, that there is something real going on, that the grown-ups are in on it, and that the grown-ups are taking care of it. This information, presented in an *honest and developmentally appropriate* way (my two linchpins of communication with children about hard things), will do much to soothe your child and, therefore, much to calm her tantrums. You can read more about this approach, and others like it, in Chapter 12.

If your toddler or preschooler has been throwing a lot of tantrums, or they've picked up in frequency, severity, or duration, and you've considered all the young-child brain factors, the parental contributions, and the family context, and yet you still can't figure out what might be triggering these little (or—sigh—not so little) explosions, ask yourself:

> "If I took my toddler's tantrums completely out of the picture and looked at our life right now, what has recently changed or feels particularly challenging?"

And that brings us right back to the crux of the matter: what your child is capable of dealing with, what stressors you're dealing with, and what you can do about them. It turns out that, regardless of the particular goings-on in your family, you have everything you need right at hand: love and limits.

So What Now?: The "L" Words

That's good news, isn't it? And this is your way into the really concrete, pragmatic sections of this book, the ones that focus on what you actually can *do* to prevent and deescalate tantrums, not only in general, but also at notoriously tricky times of day, in known tricky settings, and during various tricky circumstances. I even go one further and provide a list of things *not* to do if your goal is to prevent and deescalate tantrums (don't say I never did anything for you). So here we go: a little less conversation, a little more action (thank you, Elvis).

Decades of research demonstrate that healthy parenting—the kind that leads to healthy, well-adjusted children—involves two important dimensions, otherwise known as the "L words": love (ensuring your children feel loved—which, by the way, is subtly but critically different from loving your children) and limits (structure, rules). Although I'm simplifying an enormous amount of data, the take-home message is this: for the most part, children who grow up in homes with high levels of both structure and warmth tend to fare best in this world on a range of different outcomes. Children from homes with high structure and low warmth, or high warmth and low structure, tend not to do quite as well, and that is even more true for children whose homes provide low structure and low warmth. It turns out that if your parenting style involves equal and abundant measures of both love and limits, you're doing more than OK and many of the other details we, as parents, obsess about pale in importance.

Too often, the parents with whom I work visualize love and limits on a continuum, with love on one side and limits on the other. They assume, in other words, that when one goes up, either in a particular situation or in one's home overall, the other one needs to go down. For example, I recently met with a father who recounted a frustrating experience he'd had with his daughter, Alix, the weekend before. The two of them had passed an ice-cream cart while on an afternoon walk in Central Park, and, of course, Alix asked her dad for ice cream as soon as she saw it. She had just had a cookie, though, and her dad didn't think a second dessert was a good idea. Alix begged and pleaded with him, unable to focus on anything else. Dad held his ground and, out of ideas, finally ignored her tantrum altogether so as not to indulge her bad behavior. It was then that Alix punched her father in the thigh, leading him to put her on a park bench for a time-out (see Chapter 9 for more on time-outs and tantrums); she wailed from start to finish. The two of them then walked home, silent but for Alix's whimpers and sniffling. Her father was crushed that his precious (and somewhat rare) one-on-one time with his daughter had taken such a negative turn, and he wasn't able to see how the interaction might have gone differently—unless, of course, he had gotten Alix the ice cream, which didn't feel like the right solution.

 "Should I be giving my children time-outs when they throw tantrums? I've read so much contradictory information about this and just want to do the right thing!"

 The answer to this question is straightforward: no. The reasons behind it, however, are less so. I actually believe in time-out, although it's frustrating that I need to use the word "believe" in this context.

This is not about believing or not believing in the effectiveness of this technique; the science is very clear that, as a behavioral approach for *discrete negative behaviors*, time-outs work very well *when they are implemented correctly and as originally intended*. However, "time-out" has been misunderstood and misapplied on nearly every level, including when, how, and for what it should be used. Part of the reason for this is that it has been falsely and misleadingly placed in opposition to "time-in," a phrase that has come to be equated with providing comfort and emotional connection to children. The fact is, however, that, for the most part, everyday parenting should look like "time-in"; it is not a separate intervention unto itself. Furthermore, "time-out" works only when children are accustomed to experiencing "time-in" with their parents—when there is sufficient contrast for the "time-out" from attention (which is all it is) to be notable and, therefore, impactful. It's unfortunate, to my mind, that the controversy around time-out has been fueled more by irresponsible (if effective) marketing and less by what we know works for kids. If you want to know more about how to use time-out effectively and as informed by science, see: *https://greatergood.berkeley.edu/article/ item/six_ingredients_to_an_effective_time_out.*

All of that said, I do not want to be sidetracked by this issue because regardless of whether you use time-out in your home, the technique is not an appropriate or (more important) effective response to tantrums. Tantrums are expressions of emotion, responses to situations or feelings that children find overwhelming in some way. They might be comprised of specific behaviors, some of which may be addressed effectively with the use of time-out (for example, hitting), and some of which will not (for example, crying). When children become overwhelmed by emotion, they may benefit from some time away from you or from stimulation more generally. Allowing your child to take a break from the situation at hand, or giving him some time away to calm down, is not the equivalent of the behavioral technique of "time-out" in its strictest, and most accurate, sense. We, as professionals, owe it to you, as parents, to strive for more clarity in the language we use around this. Parenting is hard enough as it is—no need to create controversy where none need exist!

In this scenario, Alix's dad felt like he had a binary choice between love and limits, that the only way he could connect with his daughter as she was throwing a tantrum in the middle of the park was to give in and buy her an ice-cream cone. In his mind, he had only two choices: either hold firm or give in. What he neglected to see—as so many parents do—is that there was a way to provide Alix with both love and limits at the same time, because the two exist on separate axes, rather than along one continuum. Structure and warmth are not mutually exclusive and are actually most powerful when exercised simultaneously.

> Using love and limits is not a zero-sum game: applying one doesn't mean sacrificing the other.

And so, I introduced a third possibility to Alix's father: what if he were to show compassion toward Alix, to empathize that it's really hard not to get what you want when you want it, all while maintaining the limit around not getting ice cream? In other words, the word "no" doesn't have to stand alone to be effective, and showing warmth to your child doesn't have to signify your approval of her behavior. In all likelihood, Alix didn't end up hitting her father because he wouldn't buy her ice cream (in which case, she would have done so earlier in their interaction), but because she felt like her father wasn't hearing how upset she was and she needed to show him—and let out her angry feelings—in the only way she knew how in that moment. If her father had empathized with her desire for ice cream, rather than simply shutting it down, he might have been able to avoid Alix's meltdown.

Let's look at the other side of the same coin. One of the mothers with whom I work, Petra, told me in one of our sessions that she had returned home from her high-pressure job the night before and had barely gotten through the door before her son, Ari, ran toward her and wrapped his arms around her legs in a bear hug. Petra was delighted to see her little guy, but also exhausted and dying to have five minutes to exhale and change out of her suit. She gave Ari a quick, distracted hug and headed to her bedroom, letting Ari know she'd be back in a moment. Ari, of course, didn't like this plan. He collapsed to the floor, crying and kicking his legs, which led Petra to feel overcome with guilt. She quickly walked back to join Ari on the floor, where the two of them began to play Legos together. "The whole time, though," she confessed to me, "I just kept thinking about how uncomfortable I was sitting on the floor in my suit, which then made me feel ashamed because I hadn't seen Ari all day—who cares about my suit? Maybe I'll start taking a change of clothes to work, and I'll change in the bathroom there before I head home."

Petra was in a bind similar to that of Alix's father, although in the opposite direction. She was so terrified of losing her connection with Ari—of somehow sacrificing the love between them—that she failed to set a limit that really needed to be set. Because even though getting down on the floor with Ari appeased him temporarily, it's impossible for parents to go through their lives making choices with the sole purpose of preventing their children from becoming upset. Sadness, anger, and frustration are part of life; it's best that children learn that reality within a safe and loving family and home so they're not blindsided by it later on. If Petra were to continue handling Ari's distress in this manner, Ari would likely internalize two important messages over time: (1) he's in charge—if he cries or becomes angry, the world adjusts to suit his needs, and (2) his emotions *are* really as scary as it feels like they are—so scary that even the grown-ups will do anything to get them to go away. These messages can put kids on the road to unnecessary anxiety as they grow up. Beyond that, imagine the resentment Petra would come to feel after a week or two of carrying clothes to work and changing in the bathroom before she heads home!

Q "Isn't it good for kids to feel a little bit afraid of their parents? I always felt afraid of mine, and sometimes it worries me that my child seems to have no fear when I raise my voice or get angry."

A No. It's not good for children to feel afraid of their parents, really under any circumstances. By definition, feeling afraid means feeling unsafe, and when children feel unsafe with the people they're supposed to trust and rely on most (their parents/caregivers), they're at risk for a host of negative outcomes. I get it, though. I really do. In the short term, having our kids fear us is a really appealing prospect. They'd be a lot more cooperative and compliant, probably calmer and quieter, and there would be far fewer daily battles and subsequent tantrums. Sounds blissful, right? Right. In the short term. The problem, however, emerges when we take a longer view of development, because over time the constant experience of fear—even in the background—is highly stressful for children and puts them at risk for a range of emotional, psychological, and even physical problems.

"But I didn't have any of those issues!" you may be thinking. In which case, that's great to hear (truly). Whenever I cite research findings (which these are), it's important to realize that they are based on large samples, or groups, of people, not on individuals.

Saying that something (in this case, feeling unsafe with one's parents) increases one's risk for something else (in this case, various negative outcomes) does not mean that this pathway holds true for every individual. In fact, there is an enormous body of research looking at exactly this question: What accounts for individual differences in risk and resilience? In addition, we need to be really careful with the words "afraid" and "fear." They are serious words with serious connotations, and so, when we use them colloquially, it's critical to specify our meaning. If you, for example, broke a vase when you were little and were afraid of the way your parents would react because you felt guilty and hated to let them down, or knew they'd take away your dessert and you loved dessert (who doesn't?), then that's one thing. It's another thing when a child, say, lives in fear of her mother's unpredictable and, at times, aggressive rage after she has had a few drinks or a hard day at work.

What we want is for kids to know that their parents are safe, accepting, and unconditionally loving, while *also* knowing that they are clear, boundaried, predictable, and firm when needed. Embracing this combination in our parenting is the number-one thing we can do to ensure—to the extent we can—that our children thrive emotionally, socially, and with regard to school and professional achievement (really). It all goes back to the two "L" words.

And so, again, let's allow a third possibility to emerge, one that opens up when we make space for love and limits, our two "L" words, to coexist. What if Petra were to bend down when she gets home and give Ari a long and connected hug from a place of presence rather than distraction? And what if she then said something like "Mommy is so excited to see you and to play with you, and first she needs to go into her room and change her clothes"? And if—or, rather, when—Ari starts to cry? Well, then it's not about giving up the limit, but rather about maintaining it while offering warmth as well: "I know, Ari, sweetie; it can be tough when Mama comes home and can't play with you right away. I get it. I'll be back in just a few minutes." Armed with the knowledge that his mother is the boss *and also* understands how he feels, my best guess is that Ari would be able to pull himself together, tolerate his frustration, and exercise patience (even if only for a few precious moments!) until Petra came back to play Legos.

Using the "L" words—setting limits and showing love—is nothing new for parents; in fact, it's probably how you spend pretty much all day, every day. Using them both at the same time, however, is the part that can feel novel and the part that can be a real game changer when it comes to thinking about your toddler's tantrums. Because no matter how many contributing factors are at play, chances are that "upping" love, limits, or both—before, during, and after the meltdowns themselves—is at least one of the most effective "prescriptions" you'll come across. The next two chapters will tell you more about how to do just that.

6

"Of Course You'll Always Be My Sweet Little Baby (Except Possibly When You Pee in the Bath on Purpose)"

Preserving the Authentic Connection with Your Toddler

The extent to which you can reduce the frequency and intensity of your toddler's or preschooler's tantrums very much depends on not only the existence but also the strength of the love and limits in your home. (I can't say often enough that you'll never completely get rid of tantrums, because they're a normal and important part of development.) This chapter zeroes in on the first of those two dimensions, the love between you and your child. When I tell parents that one of the first things we need to do is talk about their love for their son or daughter, the relationship as it currently stands, I am typically met with responses like "Oh, don't worry; our relationship is fine," and then, within the same breath, "It's really just the tantrums that are the problem" or "I just need more tools."

I get it. And if I thought I could save you time and energy by blowing through this part and skipping to the concrete tools, I would.

Most of the time it's not that easy, which is why the first half of this book provides so much information about the complex factors involved in creating tantrums. But the relationship you have with your child is the foundation on which all else rests. It's worth a close and honest look.

Taking a Close Look at the Foundation

You may sincerely feel your relationship with your toddler or preschooler is fine, because of course you *do* love the little munchkin. In reality, though, relationships with diabolical tantrum-throwing creatures often get shaky or start feeling forced or tense in some way. If it's at all possible that this is the case for you, this is where we need to begin.

That may mean owning—saying to yourself explicitly—that you've just about had it with your kid. You can't wait until she goes off to her twos program for the day, and you're counting down until the night you have the babysitter next week so you can escape the dreaded (and now newly epic) bedtime routine. She always acts like an angel for babysitters anyway. Or you need to take a deep breath, think back, and realize that you genuinely don't remember the last time you felt your heart explode with love for your little guy. On an intellectual level, you know you adore him, but it's really hard to connect to that feeling when he's just so *annoying* so much of the time. More than anything else, you feel trapped.

I recently met with a mother for a consultation about four-year-old Declan's constant defiance and tantrums in the face of being told "no." Whenever Jackie refused to give Declan something he asked for (read: demanded)—another cookie, a second TV show, an extra story at bedtime— he went into full-on meltdown mode, screaming, kicking, sometimes even lunging and scratching. As Jackie described these interactions with her son, she spoke quickly, as though she were rushing to a certain punch line. She spoke of various strategies she had attempted—many of which were spot on, and the same recommendations I often give to my clients—all in the same somewhat frenetic tone. When she finished, she paused and took a breath. I noticed her clenched fingers and the tightness in her face. "How do you feel?" I asked.

"What do you mean?" Jackie looked puzzled.

"How do you feel, right now, right here, in this moment, having just unloaded so much of what's going on between you and Declan?" I intentionally phrased the question in this way—drawing attention to the dynamic between them—rather than focusing solely on Declan's behavior.

Jackie paused and took a deep breath. She exhaled slowly. "I guess I feel anxious."

"Yeah," I said, glad she had expressed what I too had sensed. "When you talk about all of this, you seem tense. It seems like there's a connectedness that might be missing."

Jackie teared up. She began to explain that Declan's behavior had become so bad that she didn't enjoy him at all anymore, that she didn't "get" him, that she felt so much closer to her three-year-old, which then made her feel almost unbearably guilty; she never wanted to be the "kind of mom" who so clearly preferred one child to the other. (Possible history of childhood sibling "stuff" alert!) Now we were getting somewhere, and I started to feel hopeful about our prospects for improving Declan's behavior—much more so than when she had been speaking so rapidly a few minutes earlier. Why? How could I feel hope as this poor mother talked about how distant she felt from her son? Because acknowledging these feelings outright—truly and deeply acknowledging them, which includes making space for any accompanying emotions that bubble up—is an important and necessary first step. If I'm working with a parent who can say these things, out loud, to herself and to me, I start to feel optimistic that there can be movement, that we'll be able to make real progress. If, on the other hand, I'm working with a parent who insists things are fine, yet whose tone of voice and body language suggest otherwise, I know we have an uphill climb before us.

Being Real with Yourself

By sharing Jackie's story, I'm not at all suggesting that every parent who comes to me about tantrums has reached this point, only that it's important to be honest and real with yourself if you have. Ask yourself the following questions, maybe even jotting down some notes as you go:

- What's something super cute and quirky that my child does?
- When was the last time he made me laugh (a real, genuine, from-the-belly-up laugh, not the contrived kind that you put on to humor him, as in "Ha, you put your shoe on your head instead of your foot—that's *hilarious!*")?
- What's special about my child?
- When was the last time I felt actively grateful to be the mother/father of such a sweet little cuddle nugget? What prompted this feeling?
- What was a recent moment of real connection between us, when I really "got" my child and I could tell she felt that?

Now take a moment to reflect: What was it like to answer those questions? Did the responses come naturally? Could you have said much, much more?

Did the corners of your mouth start to turn up, and did you perhaps feel a bit of warmth in your heart? If so, your connection to your child is probably in pretty good shape. Alternatively, did you struggle a bit, or feel pressured, like there were right and wrong answers? Did it feel like you were trying to "sell" your child and the relationship you have with him or her, cognizant of what the responses would look like to an outside observer? If so, then the relationship may be a bit strained and calling out for our attention.

It's the Repair That Matters

Needless to say (I hope), I know it's not quite this simple. I can't ask you to answer five questions about your toddler or preschooler, have you reflect on your experience answering them, and then jump to a sweeping conclusion about the status of your parent–child relationship. There are a host of other factors at play, and our relationships with our children are way more nuanced and complicated than that. That said, being honest with *yourself*— based on your experience with these questions or whatever other proxies you choose to draw on—is what's important here. Please note (and underline, and highlight): *regardless of where you assess your relationship with your child to be right now, it's OK.* There is no judgment here. Truly. You are exactly where you are, and exactly where you are is OK. Your relationship with your child is not stagnant, and acknowledging some, or even a lot of, strain is not a life sentence. Far from it. In fact, the idea that "rupture and repair" is not only necessary in, but beneficial to, parent–child relationships is well grounded in research. Ruptures—moments or periods of disconnection in the relationship—are both natural and inevitable. What's important is the nature of the "repair," how quickly and effectively parents and children can come back into sync and reconnect after losing each other.

> No behavioral strategy stands a chance of reducing tantrums if the parent–child relationship feels shaky.

Your child's seemingly excessive tantrums may be a sign that a repair is needed, that the two of you are out of sync and have to find each other again. Because if your relationship is ruptured, and you are as tense as Jackie was when describing her recent interactions with Declan, there is no doubt in my mind that your toddler or preschooler senses that. As we've discussed, young children are sponges, acutely aware of the emotions and energies that surround them, especially when it comes to their parents. And if your child senses a lack of connection between you, she will experience this as overwhelming, and the tantrums will continue in full force. All the behavioral strategies in the world won't begin to touch the tantrums children throw when the parent–child relationship feels broken or out of whack in some way. The relationship between you and your child is the foundation; we need to make sure that it's sturdy and strong before we even attempt to build on it by introducing new skills and strategies (yours and your child's).

Loving Our Children for Who They Are (Even When That's Not Pretty): Secure Attachment

So how do we do that? First, we have to decide what a strong and healthy relationship between a parent and child looks like. I could write a whole book—scratch that, 10 whole books—about that. Parent–child relationships that lead to positive child outcomes are typically characterized by a "secure attachment," about which I could also write 10 whole books, except I never would, because others have, and many are quite good (see the Resources, as well as the box on page 76 in Chapter 4). In short, within the framework of attachment theory—and as borne out in decades of research—parents of children who are securely attached are attuned to their children and respond to their needs in a developmentally appropriate, contingent manner. In plain English, children need to feel that their parents "get" them, that they see, accept, and love them for who they are—even when things get tough. So what does this look like exactly? Let me use a personal example.

I recently backed into a parked car. It was raining, I was doing a three-point ("K") turn on a dead-end street, and I reversed the car right into the driver's-side door of a parked sedan. I got out to examine the damage and saw that I had, in fact, left a small (OK, maybe a tiny bit bigger than small) dent. After snapping a picture and leaving a note with my contact information on the windshield, I promptly called my husband to share the news. His response? "Ugh." But it was a really heartfelt, guttural, extended "ugh," an "ugh" that I could tell, even over the phone, was accompanied by a wrinkling forehead and full stop. "Ugh" isn't even an English word, but in that one sound, I felt "gotten." Here's why. In that one syllable, I heard that my husband understood not just that fender benders are a bummer in general (anyone could get that), but that they are a particular bummer for *me*: that I've had just enough of them in my life to feel shame about my driving, that they trigger how insecure I sometimes feel about my poor visual-spatial skills (I've been known to break a glass by banging it onto the granite counter in the process of missing the sink), and that I'd likely go on to spend the rest of the day anxiously contemplating the possibility that one day I'll get into a more serious accident, maybe even with the kids in the car. My husband's "ugh" was an acknowledgment of *my* history, *my* need for compassion, in that moment. That my driving skills seem questionable to me is part of my stuff (and the stuff of Chapter 4), and in knowing that, my husband showed he got me and accepted me despite the occasional dent.

Truly "getting" someone isn't just about empathizing, although empathizing is certainly a piece of it. It's about knowing your audience. Someone else who'd just backed into a parked car might have wanted reassurance along the lines of "It's all going to be OK" or "In the grand scheme of things, a fender bender isn't such a big deal." Another person might have craved more concrete direction: "Hold on, let me get GEICO on the phone and see how much something like this might affect our premiums." In the case of parenting, "getting" your kid means understanding who *he* is—*his* history, personality, preferences, triggers, delights—and then acting in such a way that communicates your full acceptance of, and love for, that *particular* little person. Does this mean you need to understand everything about your little one? No. Or love everything about him? For sure no. Or always get along? Thankfully, a definitive NO. But to manage tantrums more effectively, you need to "get"—to know and to love—your kid overall.

> When little kids—and the rest of us—don't feel gotten, they (and we!) act out.

Why is this so important? Because when toddlers and preschoolers don't feel "gotten," they often act out. They feel anxious, misunderstood, alone, not truly seen, not accepted for who they are, or some combination of these emotions—none of which they may be able to put into words, and thus any and all of which can easily result in overwhelm and tantrums. Think about my fender bender. Upon hearing my husband's "ugh," I felt my heart rate slow, my shoulders relax, my eyes release a few cathartic tears. We were able to have a calm and connected conversation about the extent of the damage and the next steps. Had he responded in a way that didn't communicate his fully "getting" me, the following ten minutes would likely have looked quite different. I might have felt judged or misunderstood. My heart rate would have increased and my body would have tensed up. Maybe I would have stayed on the phone and gotten snippy, defensive, or accusatory ("What, *you've* never made a mistake before, Mr.

Perfect?"). Maybe I would have hung up and needed to isolate for a bit. The point is, feeling like he "got" me in that moment allowed us to connect, which then allowed me to calm down, which then allowed—after a little time had passed—us to problem-solve. The same is true for our kids.

I recently worked with parents who were concerned about the tantrums their daughter, Mia, was having every morning at preschool drop-off. These parents reached out in mid-October; it had been about a month since the beginning of school, and the tantrums were getting worse and not better. Most of the time it was Mia's mother, Pam, who brought her to school. Typically, Pam said, Mia was absolutely fine right up until they entered the building, at which point her lip would quiver, and she would, over the next minute or so, spiral into a complete meltdown, which apparently persisted until about five minutes after Pam left (according to the teacher's report). "In the beginning it was awful," Pam said to me. "It was heart wrenching. But at this point, I've tried everything, nothing works, and I know it's coming, and I just dread it and want to get it over with. Honestly, now I feel mostly irritated."

I asked Pam what exactly she had tried, observing her roll her eyes and sigh with exasperation before she responded. "I've told her that she loves school! That she's going to have a great time as soon as I leave, because she always does! And I've told her that I don't have time to do this every morning, that I have to get to work, and that my work is important for our family. And I've told her that she has to go to preschool because kids have to go to school to learn and be smart. I even told her that if she doesn't cry in the morning she can have a special snack after school, but miraculously this is the one time that hasn't made a difference!"

Pam's shoulders were high up by her ears—clearly held in tension—and her jaw was tight. I heard so much frustration in her words and so much veiled (albeit not that well) anxiety about the situation at hand. What I didn't hear was any sense of what Mia might be going through, any sign that Pam was able to "get" Mia in those difficult moments. "Would you allow me to veer from this topic for just a moment?" I asked. With her permission, I continued. "Tell me about the first time you held Mia, after she had just been born" (I knew, from my intake, that Pam's delivery had been a smooth one and that there had been no postbirth complications). Pam's whole face and energy softened as we began to speak about that first tender moment and the ones that followed. Her shoulders visibly shifted downward, and her jaw relaxed. She spontaneously took a deep breath as her nervous system clearly settled. Now that she was in a different place, I asked her to put herself in Mia's shoes. Specifically, I asked Pam to close her eyes and picture dropoff. "How do you think Mia feels when you're about to leave?"

Over the course of the conversation, Pam was able to see Mia for who she was in those moments, not a vindictive pest whose goal was to annoy her mother and make her late to work, but a scared little girl who'd never been to school before and who needed her mommy to understand her emotional experience. Within that context, Pam could also see why none of what she had tried thus far—her various explanations and attempts to put an incentive system in place—had been effective. Nothing had gotten to the heart of the matter, Mia's need to connect, in a deep and authentic way, with her mother prior to their separation. In fact, even on the occasions when Pam *had* attempted to connect—with a hug good-bye or an assurance she'd be back soon—she was likely doing so with body language and a vocal quality that signaled tension (such as stiff shoulders or jaw, a distracted, hurried, or even exasperated tone). Our children hear our words, but, even more so, they pick up on the energy behind them; Pam was going through the "right" motions, but acting from a place of emotional dysregulation, all the while waiting for the other shoe to drop. Given that, it's no surprise that Mia couldn't be soothed—and actually seemed to be further activated—by this energy. Once Pam understood what was going on, I didn't need to feed her the words to say to her daughter. In fact, just the opposite; it was as if some kind of dam had broken, and the words came pouring out of her mouth in a heartfelt and genuine way. "I have to let her know that I understand how she feels," Pam said, "and that I'm always with her during the day even if we're not physically together, and that her feelings are natural, and that I get them, and that I've had them myself when I've been in new situations. And I have to give her a huge bear hug instead of a quick, compulsory one, and I have to let her know that I can't wait to see her at the end of the day and will be thinking about her until then." All I had to do was nod. Within a week or so, Mia's meltdowns at dropoff were a thing of the past.

> We are hardwired to sense whether or not we are being seen, heard, or understood.

When we are not fully seen, heard, or understood—"gotten"—we sense it. Not because we are super smart or cognitively skilled, but because, physiologically, we're wired from birth to be social animals, designed to pick up on the extent to which others around us are safe and reliable, whether they'll be able to provide the sense of connection we are *biologically driven* to need. Our little ones know when we get them and when we don't. When we feel frustrated by them, or impatient, or puzzled in an anxious (versus open and curious) way, it's clear. Even if we attempt to be positive, empathic, or loving in our words, our bodies (in Pam's case, her stiff shoulders and jaw) and/or tones of voice give us away.

A lot of the time, our frustration and impatience are short-lived; these emotions flare up in response to something your toddler or preschooler is doing, and the connection between you is briefly ruptured. Then a repair happens—often not even consciously—and you bounce back into sync. Last night, I was ready to strangle Henry during dinner—honestly, I don't even remember why. What I do remember is that it passed when he accidentally knocked over his cup of water, but (amazingly) was able to catch it before it tipped over. He looked up at me, clearly pleasantly shocked by his own spill-avoiding prowess, and I exclaimed—without even thinking about it—"Nice move, Buddy!" Just like that, we were back to good. Episodes like these happen *all the time* with our little ones—multiple times per day—and, as mentioned above, have been shown to be essential for healthy early childhood development. It's when parents' periods of frustration become more prolonged that a cycle can begin in which the ruptures far outnumber the repairs and the tantrums pick up in frequency and intensity. It's during these cycles that particular care must be given to get the parent–child relationship back on track (or, sometimes, on track in the first place).

Three Steps You Can Take to Reconnect

And so if, after some honest and deep reflection, you can say that you are currently feeling connected to, like you "get," your little one, and your toddler knows and feels it, that's fantastic; you're ready to move on from this chapter. That said, please don't forget about it; relationships with our children ebb and flow, and just because things feel solid right now doesn't mean they always will. If you're reading this in actual book form, consider dog-earing or putting a Post-It on this page so that you can return to it easily, both literally and symbolically. If you're using an e-reader, add a highlight. That is to say: when in doubt—about how to manage tantrums or, frankly, any other difficult behavior you see in your child over the next few years—return to the relationship as a starting point. It really is that foundational.

And if, after honest and deep reflection, this is not where you're at right now—you're not feeling like you're connected and really "get" your kid—that's OK too. Why? Two reasons. First, because again, we're not judging. You are where you are, and wherever you are—especially if you acknowledge and accept it—is OK. Second, because there are things we can do about it. There are active steps you can take to strengthen and deepen your relationship with your little one—starting today. Making a commitment to do this, and following through on it, is the first and by far most important action you can take to decrease the frequency and intensity of your child's tantrums.

Here are three approaches to try. (Note: if you are beyond giving these suggestions a shot—if you skim the following paragraphs and notice yourself rolling your eyes, assuming they're pretty much worthless—there's no judgment there either. Truly, this whole book is a judgment-free zone. What there may be, however, is some evidence to suggest that you could benefit from seeking out professional guidance, in the form of an individual or dyadic [parent–child] therapist who can do a thorough assessment to determine what's not working in your relationship with your child, and formulate a plan for addressing it. See the Resources for more information on how to do this.)

1. *Go look at pictures of your kid as a baby.* Sound cheesy? Yeah, it is a little. But effective. The picture of when you first brought your newborn home from the hospital? Or the first time the dog went over to sniff her out? Or the one from her first birthday when her face and both hands are covered in chocolate frosting? And the videos! Don't forget about the videos! When your child first started babbling and you recorded the in-depth "conversation" you had? Or when he was first learning to walk and had that adorable, proud grin as he tottered toward the camera? The one where your little girl has that infectious, gurgling giggle? When we see certain photographs and videos of our children, we can't help smiling and feeling a warmth rise up in our hearts. Go spend some time with your favorites—not hours, but not mere seconds either. Sit somewhere comfortable, take out some albums, or your computer/phone/tablet, and let yourself get carried away.

2. *Do a visualization or writing exercise about some of the most amazing moments you've had with your child to date.* Do you remember when she first smiled at you? Or called you Mama or Dada? Said she loved you? Or reached up for you from the crib? Or when you took him swimming for the first time? Or got in a tickle fight? Or when he last put his head on your shoulder after a nap? Or fell asleep on your lap when he had a fever?

Choose a memory that feels poignant for you and spend some time with it. Think—or write—about what happened, using as many details—and sense memories—as possible. What did your child's skin feel like against yours in the ocean? What did his sweaty hair feel like under your palms when he had a fever? What was he wearing when he first said "Mama"? What did she smell like when you buried your head in her tummy and tickled her?

And if, as you do this, some negative feelings come up for you—"Ugh, right now the sound of her giggle just grates on me"—just let them be there, rather than trying to push them away. The only way to feel connected again is to be authentic; again, it's the authenticity that allows for the movement. If, for example, as you slow down the memory of your daughter first saying "I love you," you find yourself thinking, "She hasn't said that in a while; I wonder if she still does," just let yourself feel that. See what happens. We have to be present—with our whole selves—to be wholly present with our kids.

3. *Start implementing "Special Mommy" and/or "Special Daddy" time.* Research shows that spending even just five or ten minutes a day with your young child—and intentionally referring to the time as "Special Mommy and Ryan" or "Special Daddy and Charlotte" time—can do a lot to strengthen the parent–child relationship and, in turn, decrease disruptive behaviors. Doing special time this way—a little bit each day—has actually been shown to be more effective toward these ends than planning, say, a whole day's outing or adventure together every couple of weekends. Special time becomes part of the daily routine and is not dependent or contingent on your little one's behavior. This way the message becomes one of unconditional acceptance rather than "I only spend time with you when you're good." Ideally, your child chooses the activity, and it's one you can engage in together (reading, coloring, a board game, playing outside, building with blocks). The idea—and priority—is to enjoy each other, have fun together. No criticizing or commands allowed. Make it connected; maybe even make a mess.

You Are Your Toddler's Safe Person

There's a reason so many parents tell me their toddlers and preschoolers behave like angels when they're at school, with the nanny/babysitter, or with their grandparents. I've heard it time and time again: "I just don't get it! Everyone says he's the sweetest little angel when I'm not there, but once I'm around, he morphs into a terror!" If this is you, it might be easy to assume that the reason is a rupture within the parent–child relationship. After all, if you're the person he acts out with the most, then you must be the person with whom he has the biggest problem, right? Wrong. There's actually another, more common possibility, which is the one I want to highlight as this chapter comes to a close. You are your child's safe person. The one she knows she can lose it around. The one she knows isn't going anywhere, no matter what she throws at you (literally and figuratively). The one she trusts she can just *be* with—letting her toddler or preschooler brain do whatever it's going to do—without having to *act* in any particular way or *do* anything extra. Is this a conscious choice your toddler or preschooler makes? Of course not. It's just something we innately know, and then continue to learn as we grow, about where and with whom it's safe to show all aspects of ourselves versus only the good parts. We put forth our true colors and let our freak flags fly when we feel like someone loves us, and will never stop loving us, exactly as we are. That's what a secure attachment looks like.

Toddlers and preschoolers need to hear this message—*I get you*—over and over again. They also need to hear its complement: *I've got you*. That is, not only do I see and love you, but I can *contain* you; you are not too big for me. The next chapter moves on from "I get you" to "I've got you," from love to limits.

7

"Who's Making the Rules Here?"

Using Reasonable Structures and Routines to Help Your Toddler Feel Secure

When we're at the end of our rope with our child's tantrums, it's easy to assume the problem is that we're being too soft, too permissive. So let's get one misconception out of the way right now: when I talked about "containing" your child at the end of Chapter 6, I wasn't talking about punishment or that children should be seen and not heard. In a general sense, I meant helping your little ones know where they fit within this big, seemingly chaotic world and that you're there to keep things from getting overwhelmingly out of control. I also talked about love before getting to limits for a good reason: Any attempt to impose structure and routine for your toddler or preschooler will be infinitely more effective within the context of an authentic, accepting connection. So even though I hope you'll take to heart the message from Chapter 5 that children do best with love and limits provided in equal measure, if you need to focus on one before the other, I recommend (based on a vast research literature) that you make addressing any shakiness in the parent–child relationship your first priority. Ultimately, the idea is to be able to set limits while maintaining a connection to your kids, or—conversely—to love your kids madly within the context, or container, of an overarching structure.

There's Safety in Predictability

Love is important (among other things!) because when children know it's safe to be exactly who they are, the overwhelming frustration, anxiety, or general upset that can lead to tantrums is minimized. Limits are important when it comes to preventing tantrums because children feel safer when limits are in place. When I give presentations, I often use a graphic I found online (I'd be happy to give more specific credit, but it doesn't seem to exist) in which a little baby is sitting comfortably within a light-blue rectangle drawn around him. Around the border of the rectangle are the words "Discipline is a boundary inside which your children feel secure and loved." Discipline, therefore, or limits—my preferred term—is neither intended nor designed to be punitive in nature. Rather, limits are meant to delineate a safe space in which children can feel clear on expectations and predict certain structures and routines. This is why I like to use the word "container" when talking about the role that limits play for young children. The emotions and behavior of toddlers and preschoolers might be all over the place, given how exciting, fun, stimulating—and, at times, overwhelming and scary—the world looks through young eyes and rapidly developing brains. But when children feel contained—when they understand what's going on and can predict what's coming next—they are less likely to feel anxious, overwhelmed, or frustrated, all emotional experiences that increase the likelihood of tantrums.

> **Limits help children feel safe, secure, and loved.**

The same is true for adults. Think about the last time you weren't quite sure which way was up. It may have been your first day at a new job, or in a new house or apartment, or even just a new supermarket. In each of these situations—to different extents for different people—we get a bit nervous, we feel somehow off our game. Why? At least in part because we don't yet know the routine, the norms, how things work, what goes where. At the new job: Do people leave their doors open in this office? How does the email system work? Who keeps track of my sick days? In the new house: What drawer is the silverware in again? Why can't I find my favorite black pants? I keep going right instead of left to get to the bathroom! In the supermarket: They put the bananas here? Seriously? Why on earth would they put the bananas here? And where's the Pirate's Booty section?

When we can't find our bearings, we start to feel a bit tense—our heart rates may increase, our blood pressure may go up, we become irritable or sensitive as we work to orient ourselves. Let's do a quick exercise. Picture yourself at your local airport. You're supposed to board a plane that takes off at 9:40 A.M., which means that, according to your ticket and the TV monitor on the wall, boarding is set to begin at 9:10 A.M. You got to the gate at 8:30 A.M., coffee and muffin in hand, with time to spare. It's now 9:05 A.M., so you're expecting boarding will begin any minute. You wait patiently. You look at the clock on the wall, then at your phone, then back up at the clock. It's 9:12, and still no boarding announcement. You start to pace a little. You look at your watch. It's 9:15, so you walk over to the flight attendant behind the desk and inquire about boarding. "Should be soon," he responds with a smile. You look at the clock, your phone, and your watch. It's 9:20. The flight is supposed to take off in 20 minutes. You check your email. Facebook. Instagram. Twitter. You look at your watch again: 9:24. You walk back over to the desk: "Any news?" The flight attendant shakes his head, distractedly. Now it's almost 9:27. Email. Facebook. Instagram. Twitter. It's 9:30.

Pause.

How do you feel right about now? Agitated, right? Think about what your heart rate would be doing and what your mood would be like. Let me put you out of your misery: finally—*finally*—at 9:30, the flight attendant announces that the boarding process is about to begin, that passengers should start to gather their belongings. It has been only 20 minutes—20 minutes!—since you expected to hear this announcement, and yet you feel as though you have experienced a massive delay. When a fellow passenger accidentally bumps you with his rollaboard, you feel like you could rip his head off with your bare hands (although you exercise enormous restraint and merely force a we-both-know-I'm-annoyed smile in his direction).

Now compare that scenario with this one: Again, you're at your local airport. Once again, you're supposed to board a plane that takes off at 9:40 A.M., which means that boarding is set to begin at 9:10. You got to the gate at 8:30, coffee and muffin in hand, with time to spare. It's 9:05, so you're expecting boarding will begin any minute. You wait patiently. At 9:10, the flight attendant announces that there is a slight delay and that boarding will begin in approximately 20 minutes.

Pause.

How do you feel? A bit annoyed, sure. Delays are never fun. But you're not agitated, correct? You're not anxious. You can stay in your seat, maybe even read one article, or stick to one social media platform on your phone. Why? Because you were alerted as to what's to come, you are able to predict what is going to happen next, and you know exactly when it will be happening. When Mr. Rollaboard bumps into you several minutes later as you make your way into line, you're able to smile genuinely and say "no worries"—and mean it.

When I present these two scenarios to parents, there's often an "aha" moment. They recognize the vast impact that the announcement of the delay, compared to no announcement at all, would have on both their internal state and, in turn, their behavior toward others. A few parents, of course, have pointed out that they'd feel anxious or agitated either way, but when I've probed, the responses have always been similar in nature. Specifically, these parents say things like "I know by now that one delay always leads to another" or "I've learned not to trust any airport announcements ever!" or "I only have faith the plane is taking off when I'm actually in the air." These reactions reveal a history of flying, of so much experience with the unpredictability of air travel that only actions (actual take-off versus the verbal promises of announcements) are meaningful.

> When toddlers can trust in their environment— predict what's coming and understand how things work— tantrums are less likely to erupt.

So, how does this all relate to our kids? Your children's internal states (which lay the groundwork for tantrums) and external behavior (tantrums themselves) are greatly influenced by the extent they can predict what's to come, understand how things work, trust in their environments. You, as an adult in the airport, have learned how to manage your anxiety and agitation— pacing, checking the time, and bouncing around on your phone are all coping mechanisms for channeling your anxiety and/or irritation. For all of the reasons discussed in Chapter 3, young children haven't yet developed these capacities, and so they are going to experience their feelings of anxiety or agitation as completely overwhelming. And, as always, once we have young children feeling overwhelming emotions, we have young children throwing tantrums.

A Day in the Life of Your Toddler: Routine or Not?

When talking to clients about their children's tantrums, I always—*always*— ask to be walked through the daily routine, a "day in the life" of the toddler or preschooler in question. I want to know what time the child wakes up and how breakfast typically goes. I want to know if the child is in a day care or preschool program and, if so, who does dropoff and pickup and at what times. I want to know what meals are like, what the bedtime routine is, whether baths happen every day, how many books are read before lights out. Now, I am not expecting parents to answer me as if they're running a military school—"dropoff at day care is at oh-seven-hundred hours, MA'AM!"—but I do hope to see that there is somewhat of a predictable routine, on which the child (as well as, let's face it, the parents) can rely. If there isn't, then right there is a very big clue about what's behind the tantrums.

When the Predictable Becomes Unpredictable

Often it's the case that tantrums increase when there *was* a predictable routine that has somehow been derailed, whether due to traveling, having house guests, or moving from one home to another; whether due to a new sibling, a change in nanny, or any number of other possibilities. In these cases, my advice is almost always to get back in a routine as quickly as possible and see what happens to the tantrums once the structure is reestablished (frequently, they decrease in both frequency and intensity).

Less Structure → More Meltdowns

Another frequent scenario is that tantrums typically occur at a particular time of day, and, lo and behold, it's the time of day that's least structured. Recently some clients of mine were puzzled as to why their children (ages two and four) were throwing so many tantrums in the morning when it was time to get dressed and leave the house. In contrast, the kids were great at the end of the day, from dinner all the way through bedtime. At first I was surprised; often it's the end of the day that's hardest, when everyone is tired, and so emotional reserves run low. A quick conversation, though, revealed what was going on. Namely, the nighttime routine ran like clockwork—both parents were always home, their roles were clearly defined, the whole thing was a well-choreographed dance. The morning was no such *Swan Lake*. Sometimes Dad was home to help, and other times he needed to leave early for work. Sometimes Mom had time to sit with the kids for breakfast; other times she let them watch a show while they ate so that she could shower and get ready. Sometimes the four-year-old was allowed to pick out her clothes, other times she was told what to wear. Once I had learned all of this, I hypothesized that the disorganized and unpredictable feel of the morning was likely anxiety provoking for the kids, particularly the older one, who was more sensitive to these variables (because, as always, there are individual differences when it comes to how our children respond). Furthermore, less structure means more opportunities for power struggles, and there's nothing like a solid power struggle to kick off a good tantrum.

In the case of this family, we implemented several techniques—all of which are described at the end of this chapter—that brought a higher level of structure and thus *containment* to the morning time. I want to highlight one in particular here, because it speaks to a common, and potentially damaging, misunderstanding. Specifically, when I first began working with the family, Dad told me how much it hurt his feelings in the morning when Hayley, the four-year-old, threw a tantrum upon hearing that he—rather than Mom—would be the one to drop her off at school. Once I provided information about the various reasons that tantrums are a normal part of early childhood development, and how, as parents, we cannot take these expressions of emotion personally (see Chapter 3, Chapter 9, and the Q&A at the end of Chapter 4), I asked for more information. It turned out that Dad's taking Hayley to school was a relatively rare occurrence—usually only once, occasionally twice, a week—and he did what he could to frame it as a special treat for her, a chance to spend quality time together. Instead, though, he told me that Hayley's lower lip would start quivering and inevitably she'd sit down right where she was and "pitch a fit."

As usual, I applied the lens of "love and limits" to diagnose, or better understand, the scenario this father was describing. Was there a problem in the relationship between Hayley and her dad? No, none that I observed. Did she not want to be alone with him for some reason? No, she loved when they spent time alone together in the evenings. I kept coming up blank in that category, and so I turned my focus to "limits." What if the issue was not in the relationship between Hayley and her dad, but in the lack of predictability with regard to who would take her to school in the morning? What if, I asked, there was a way for Hayley to know in advance who would be taking her to school on a particular day? What if Hayley's parents could let her know the night before, or—better yet—what if there was a schedule, preferably posted somewhere, that showed (using pictures, as Hayley couldn't yet read) whether Mom or Dad would take her to school each morning of the coming week? Sure enough, as soon as Hayley's parents implemented the latter, Hayley not only stopped crying upon learning her father would be taking her to school but actually looked forward to it. Yup, it turned out that her reaction had nothing to do with how she felt about her father, but was rather the reaction of a kid who simply needed to know a bit more about what she could expect each morning.

Playing with Surprises to Teach Resilience

Of course, this anecdote invites the question: When it comes to predictability, how much is too much? Is there such a thing as going overboard? Aren't we, as parents, trying to foster flexibility and adaptability in our little ones? The response to all three questions is yes. And yet that's where the simple answers end. As discussed in Chapter 3, where there's a whole section devoted to the rigidity of toddlers and preschoolers, we need to understand and accept this normal facet of their development, so that, when needed, we can put limits on it in an appropriate and attuned manner.

No one wanted Hayley to learn that any change in routine was intolerable, and, in fact, evidence-based treatments for children with anxiety disorders incorporate deliberate exposure to "unexpected" events (such as a restaurant running out of your favorite dessert) to foster coping skills. And yet, at the same time we also need to understand just how much of the world seems overwhelming to little minds and to help children by imposing structures that help them make sense of things when, and where, they can.

How do we know where to draw this line? As usual, unfortunately there's no formula to apply. We need to tune in to our individual kids and rely somewhat on our instincts to let us know when we have found the appropriate balance. And as is typical when it comes to parenting, right when we find it, and are reveling in our awesome instincts, something will happen and we'll need to find it all over again.

> There's no formula to help you determine how much to protect your child from the unexpected. Trust your instincts and your knowledge of your child.

There is, however, one tip I used with Hayley that may be useful here. After all, there were times when Hayley's parents didn't know in advance who would take her to school on a given morning, and it was important to "prepare" for those as well. And so, about once a week, they put a question mark on the weekly calendar instead of a picture of Mom or Dad; this meant that the school dropper-offer would be revealed only that morning. This ended up being extremely effective; not only did the question mark warn Hayley of unpredictability ahead, but it also turned the not knowing into a bit of a guessing game or mystery. What was once a possible source of anxiety became an opportunity for play, which had the added benefit of highlighting an incredibly useful way of coping with challenges, or anxiety, more generally.

And then, of course, there were the mornings when Mom or Dad needed to unexpectedly pinch hit for the other—a work emergency, coffee spilled all over a suit jacket, a migraine, and so forth. Again, Hayley's parents handled these last-minute switches playfully—"OK, guys, there has been a change of plans. Who's up for the challenge?"—thereby modeling the importance of rolling with the punches with a positive attitude (they even came up with a family cheer for such occasions).

The Structure of Consistent Expectations

Of note, day-to-day structures and routines are only one type of "limits" that are key to reducing the frequency and intensity of tantrums. The other has to do with the limits, or expectations, that surround behavior in a particular family or home. In other words, is there an understanding of and *consistent* agreement on what's OK and what's not OK? A former colleague used to reference a system she had in her home of labeling certain expectations or rules as "single Ns" or "double Ns"—negotiables or nonnegotiables, which I always thought was a catchy way to capture the idea that certain rules or expectations may be more flexible than others, but that there needs to be transparency among all members of a family about this. Because of where they are in their development with regard to seeking autonomy (as described in Chapter 3), it's the *job* of toddlers and preschoolers to test limits, to push up against them as hard as they can and see if they'll buckle or maybe even come crashing down. And, therefore, it's the job of parents to build limits that are strong and steady enough to withstand that kind of pressure. Because, again, the point is to create a boundary inside which young children feel safe and loved—feel that *we've got them.* If the boundaries come crashing down under pressure, that space cannot be created effectively.

> It's not too early to establish the difference between negotiables and nonnegotiables.

Whenever I'm talking to a parent about tantrums, I am careful to listen for certain language, phrases like "he makes me" or "she won't let me." For example, "Simon makes me sit with him until he falls asleep" or "Layla doesn't let me pick up her baby sister unless I pick her up first." Why do these phrases catch my attention so quickly? Because they suggest to me that there has been a role reversal, that parents are allowing the child to be in charge, rather than vice versa. In addition, this language often signifies parents who have come to fear their children's tantrums, who are, as many clients describe it, "walking on eggshells." It's not that these children "won't let" parents act in a certain way—a way that inevitably involves setting a limit—but that they "won't let" them do it *without getting upset.* Toddlers and preschoolers can't, in actuality, *make* parents do anything (they're only around three feet tall, after all), unless the alternative—the ensuing tantrum—is so aversive to parents that it's perceived as coercive (and effectively so!).

Limits Don't Just Help Parents— Our Kids Want Them Too

Toddlers and preschoolers *want* you to set limits. Really. Through all that yelling and screaming and crying and melting down, they're secretly hoping—albeit likely not in a conscious way—that you'll toe the line and let them know you're in charge. Because remember (I can't emphasize this enough): creating and sticking to a boundary will help them feel safe and loved. Think about the 15-year-old who doesn't have a curfew. He goes out to a party with all of his friends on a Saturday night, then watches as, one by one, they all leave because they need to get home by a certain time. As his friends go, he plays it off like he's psyched: bummer for them that they have to go home to Mommy and Daddy while he gets to stay out and rage! After his friends are all gone, though? When no one's looking, and he doesn't have to save face anymore? That kid wishes he had a curfew too.

Rules—limits— tell our kids that we care about where they are, what they're doing, and **how** they're doing.

Why? Because a curfew—a nonnegotiable limit on how late it's OK to stay out—means that someone cares when you get home; it's a rule that allows for and then *contains* exploration and autonomy, thus helping teenagers feel safe and loved.

The curfew analogy goes a long way with parents who don't actually believe their little ones want and appreciate limits, given their frequently elaborate and extensive protests to the contrary. Typically, it's enough to get parents to trust me and to at least dip their toes into settling some limits at home to see whether this has an effect on their child's tantrums (it almost always does). Before sending parents into battle, however, I arm them with one other favorite analogy, this one aimed at helping them tolerate their child's inevitable distress when limits are first imposed: Imagine your 12-year-old comes home and tells you that she is going to start smoking cigarettes and that she'd like you to buy her a pack, since she's underage. Her friends have started smoking, she thinks it's cool, and she wants in. What do you say? Parents never hesitate on this. Inevitably, they respond that they would never, ever agree to buy their daughter her first smokes. What if your daughter got mad at you? Yelled at you? Cursed at you, screamed, stormed up to her room, slammed the door? Would you buy her cigarettes then? The answer is always no. No matter how upset their future fictional 12-year-old becomes, parents are able to stick to their convictions because of their awareness that smoking is unhealthy and that their child's health and development take precedence over her anger and distress that they are laying down the law.

It is at this point that I say: ding ding ding! Because the same principle holds for toddlers and preschoolers. You are parents, you are in charge, and it is OK for you to set rules for your children—their emotional reactions, although valid and important (as reiterated in various places throughout this book), are not the measure of whether a limit or an expectation is important or valuable. And though the link between an absence of limits and an increase in tantrums may not be as clear or well documented (or, thankfully, dire) as that between smoking and lung cancer, it is, in fact, there.

Prepare for the Extinction Burst

Two final points to make before I give you some strategies for putting in place structures, routines, and limits within your home. First, the less fun one: don't be surprised if your child's tantrums get worse after the imposition of limits before they get better. In behavioral psychology, this is referred to as an extinction burst, which basically means that, if your child is used to getting what she wants by throwing a tantrum—this is how she "makes" you do something—she will simply assume that, if this is no longer the case, she just needs to try harder. That trying harder means a longer, more intense, and—from your perspective—more miserable tantrum. Until, that is, she realizes that her efforts are not paying off. It's critical that you stick with the approach until this point. Just remember, if there were no circumstance under which you would give in and buy her those cigarettes, then sooner or later she would stop cursing you out. It just may, and usually does, take a little time for your child to truly get that there's a new boss—again, a new boss she actually really *wants* to show up—in town.

Firm Rules Can Be Bent—But Handle with Care!

The second point is more fun. Namely, once structures and routines and limits are clear and in place, sturdy and strong as can be—then and *only* then—you can bend them. Young children need to know, with certainty, that we've got them, that there is a solid container in place that will hold them when their behavior or emotional reactions feel, and become, too big or out of control. Once they are equipped with this knowledge and have internalized it to some extent (which happens naturally over time), it's OK to show them that once in a while the walls may stretch or bend a bit. Which is why, case in point, my kids are allowed to have whatever they want—including cookies or ice cream (with sprinkles!)—for breakfast on their birthdays. And typically they only ask to have these absurd treats on the two or three following mornings, which I put in the victory column (because, I have to say, the size of their chocolate-smudged grins makes the yearly ritual 100% worthwhile).

Tips for Creating Structure and Routine

As you think about the importance of firming up the limits in your home, here are some guidelines/suggestions. Of note, this is an area where the age of your child makes a significant difference with regard to the approaches you choose to employ. Is your child closer to two versus three or four years old? Keep in mind your child's language and cognitive skills as you play with how to incorporate any (or all) of the following recommendations.

1. *Make a daily schedule for your home and hang it somewhere your children can see it.* As most (albeit not all) children in this age range can't read, use pictures. These can either be actual photographs (children love pictures of themselves—snap some on your phone and print them out), pictures you cut out of magazines or catalogs, or cartoons you find online. There are also, of course, various apps and websites that can assist with this. With little, tantrum-prone kiddos, ensuring regular meal and snack times, as well as a developmentally appropriate bedtime, is key, given the incredibly important role that hunger and sleep play at this age. (If you need a reminder of that, review the discussion of tantrum triggers in Chapter 2.) The schedule outlines the general order (versus exact times) of events in your home (for example, dinner, then bath, then PJs, then brushing teeth,

then stories, then song, then bedtime), so that children have a way to visualize the important routines as they internalize them.

Often, when I make this suggestion, parents assure me that their child understands the routine but that struggles frequently emerge regardless: "Oh, Xavier *knows* the morning routine, trust me; it's the same every single day. *That* is not the problem." When I ask these parents, however, how many times they prompt their child, say, in the course of a morning, that it's time to brush teeth, no one ever says "never" or even "once or twice." Most of the time, it's between four and eight times and sometimes in the double digits! The point of having a visual reminder of the routine on the wall somewhere isn't necessarily whether your child *knows* what to do next, but rather how often you need to remind him of it, thus providing the opportunity for a power struggle. Fewer reminders = less nagging (which, let's be honest, is how your child experiences your well-intentioned "reminders") = decreased likelihood that your child will experience you as the teacher in *Peanuts*: "Wah wah wah wah . . ." Although you can't stop your verbal nagging—er, I mean, prompting—the moment the pictures are on the wall, you can slowly phase it out as you point to the pictures instead. Being playful and making a game of it—"Hmm, what do we do next? I don't remember! Can you go check our schedule?"—can also do a lot to decrease tension and increase your toddler's or preschooler's sense of autonomy.

2. *Come up with some house expectations, ideally, no more than two or three—the big ones.* I prefer the word "expectations" to "rules" (although there's certainly nothing wrong with the latter), because when we're talking about young children, we're talking about creating a culture in which there are certain expectations, but not one in which we, as parents, assume these will be met flawlessly, day in and day out. I have found that when parents talk about "rules" for this age group, they—often without even realizing it—become frustrated or disappointed when their children break those rules, and then they attribute an intentionality to this transgression that isn't there.

When I say "come up with," this is as much for your sake as it is for your child's, as it's an important area in which to be thoughtful and intentional. If you are in a two-parent family, then it's also a helpful (even necessary) conversation for you to have with your partner. What behaviors are most important to you? What are the ones you can let slide? Most of the time, my clients agree that, say, "no hitting" (or other physical aggression) may be a good expectation to set, but they may disagree about whether children should be expected not to stand up on the furniture. So long as you keep in mind where your child is developmentally, and whether the expectations you set may be more about your own "stuff," there's really no right or wrong answer—so long as you're clear and consistent.

This is an area where it can also be a good idea to collaborate with your child's day care or preschool (if there is one). Find out what their expectations are and how they're communicated to the kids. After all, when a child's world is predictable (in this case, across settings), the frequency and intensity of tantrums go down. If and when you can, it's helpful to be specific and concrete (for example, "Use kind words" instead of "Be respectful"), and to phrase expectations in the positive ("Gentle hands" instead of "No hitting"). And for the umpteenth time, "No tantrums" cannot be an expectation, since tantrums are a normal and expected part of your child's development. This would be like telling your children that they're not allowed to have or show their feelings! Again, consider writing down the rules and/or illustrating them with pictures and hanging them in different places within your home. This will both communicate their importance to your child and serve as a visual reminder.

The process of coming up with expectations and then writing/posting them can be a wonderful one in which to involve your child at a level that's developmentally appropriate. Maybe your child is old enough to help come up with the content of expectations, or to decorate the rules with glitter and stickers, or help decide where to hang them. This can be a team endeavor—a wonderful way to blend love and limits and to show (both to your child and to yourself!) that the two can be, and are, intricately connected.

3. *Start having family meetings or "check-ins."* It's never too soon to start doing this. Even if your two-year-old is a bit too young to participate, the pattern is a really nice one to put in place. When having family meetings or check-ins is just a regular thing you do, they can represent a fun and connected time rather than a serious occasion implying that something's not going well (often the time when families decide to have meetings). A family—with any number of people—functions best when it's a cohesive unit, a team. A weekly or biweekly check-in, then, is a time for "teammates" to talk about what's going well and what could be going better. You might talk about how you'd like the morning hours, from wake-up through leaving the house, to be calmer, and you can brainstorm together about how to make that happen. Your four-year-old might say she'd like the kitchen to have more things that are pink in it, so you can talk about where you could

hang a pink cardboard flower she'll make for that purpose. The idea is that everyone has a voice. You can also review what the schedule holds in the week ahead, what big events are coming up, and the like. Provide popcorn or other snacks. Start by each saying something you love about everyone at the table. End with a family cheer you all make up. Someone can take notes, because even little kids who can't read understand that this makes things more "official." Family meetings are a time to reflect, to strategize, to work together—the process is as important as, if not more than, the content. Having a structure, and accompanying positive associations, in place for prioritizing communication as a family can only be a good thing as children grow.

4. *Understand that it's OK to use a firm tone of voice, which is distinct from a loud or yelling tone of voice.* When setting limits, the goal is the three "C"s: be clear, calm, and connected. This is a really important point, so let's go through the "C"s one at a time.

- *Clear*: A clear limit looks different for a toddler or preschooler than it does for an older child or adult. Although the two are not exactly synonymous, I find that a helpful shortcut is: be short. That is, use fewer words. Young children's receptive language skills are in the process of developing, and even if they're quite advanced when your child is calm, this is not the case once she becomes frustrated or upset. So often, I see parents attempting to have sophisticated discussions with their children when attempting to set a limit, using detailed explanations or extensive negotiations. More often than not, these techniques, while well intentioned, confuse young children, who really just want to be contained with a clear (read: brief) message. (More on this in the dos and don'ts suggested in Chapters 8 and 9.) Set your limit in as few words as possible and then stop talking. Simple phrases that adults could experience as condescending or strangely direct—"Please walk," "Speak softer," "Gentle hands," "Get down"—are helpful and even soothing for young children. By all means, say please, and by all means talk about the reason for a particular limit (such as safety) at another time. But in the moment that you need to set the limit, clear—short and direct—is best.

- *Calm*: Setting limits with young children is most effective when you communicate that you are both confident and at ease. Again: you've *got* this; you've *got them*. Yelling tends not to work particularly well, nor does acting as though you're calm while nonverbally communicating anxiety or overwhelm. As discussed in Chapter 6, children can sniff out inauthenticity a mile away. Being calm means exactly that: being calm. Acting calm won't cut it. There is always time— unless there's an imminent safety concern, of course (your toddler's hand an inch from the stove and moving fast)—to take a swift deep breath, feel your feet on the ground, or say a quick mantra to yourself to stay regulated (see Chapter 4).

- *Connected*: One of the most common mistakes parents make when they set limits is that they end up positioning themselves as somehow "against" their child rather than on their team. Phrases like "You see? That's what happens when . . ." or "Yup, that's what you get" or "Really? That's how you want to play this?" communicate— even if only in the moment of conflict—a sense of hostility and that you're somehow there to test and judge your child rather than protect and root for him. Parents often respond this way when they inadvertently take some behavior of their child's personally.

Let's say your child is jumping on the bed, and you're concerned he's going to fall and hurt himself. He continues to jump, despite your repeated admonitions. A message of "Just wait, you're going to hurt yourself" or "You have it coming" won't be helpful and may—and often does—increase your child's desire to prove you wrong (thus increasing the likelihood he *will* fall and hit his head). It also won't make him want to listen to you in the future, because—as discussed in Chapter 6—we listen to people who have our backs, whom we trust like us and know we're doing our best. What to say instead? "Sit on the bed, please. I *know* you can do it." Clear, calm, connected. Of course, there are a lot of other, more creative approaches you could employ as well, which is exactly the focus of the next chapter.

8

"OK. But. Now. What. Exactly. Should. I. *Do?*"

Practical Strategies for Preventing and Deescalating Tantrums

Everything discussed so far provides an essential foundation for preventing and deescalating tantrums, and if you read Chapters 1–7 you've probably already come up with some practical strategies of your own. Gaining a deeper understanding of child development, grappling with your own stuff, and addressing any important systemic or environmental issues naturally lights the way to what we can do *right now* to head off that brewing meltdown or dial back a tantrum in progress. As I've said many times, however, tantrums *will* happen. Which means you need all the tricks and tactics you can get. The following pages offer a collection of *dos* to be sure to add to your repertoire; Chapter 9 provides a list of *don't*s that are just as important.

There are essentially four different points or time periods when you can intervene most effectively in your child's tantrums, and so this chapter is divided into four sections based on the "tantrum timeline":

1. Every day, on an ongoing basis

2. Right before a tantrum begins

3. During a tantrum

4. After a tantrum

These "points of entry" are not always discrete or mutually exclusive, of course. They are an organizing device to help you think about and structure an overall plan for tantrum reduction—what you can do as a matter of course to discourage tantrums, how you can head one off that you see coming, concrete tactics for calming your child and defusing a tantrum in progress, and some "cleanup" steps you can take that will help reduce the incidence of future tantrums. In real life, these points in time can overlap, as can the recommended strategies; a technique that stops a brewing tantrum from becoming a full-blown one may also result in fewer tantrums over time if implemented in a more ongoing way.

Ongoing, Foundational Strategies to Use Every Day

You might say (or I might) that you already have a foundation for tantrum prevention if you've read Chapters 1–7. If you haven't had a chance to read them in full yet, turn to the chapters referenced in the following pages for more information. Meanwhile, here are some important overarching strategies that will support your more specific efforts.

Remember That It Rests with You

You already know this. You're the parent. And with all that's on your plate as a responsible adult, the last thing you need to hear is that *you're* the one who needs to be on your game. And yet, if you've gotten to this point in life, for better or worse (and kind of both?), adulting is mandatory. Which means you can probably use these *dos* as gentle reminders.

👍 *DO tap your creativity.*

At the end of a long, hard day you may not think you have any to offer. In the middle of a rushed supermarket trip on the way home from day care you might feel far too scattered to use your imagination. But sometimes you simply have to be able to think on your feet to find an entry point and the right strategy to defuse a simmering tantrum. This chapter is laid out along the "tantrum timeline" to give you some cues as reminders of what might work when. But be prepared to try things you haven't tried before, to play with a strategy, to give it a twist, to mix things up. When toddlers are building to the exploding point, surprise can be your friend. I wrote "The

Patience Song" (to the tune of "Where Is Thumbkin?") one evening when I would have sworn my creative juices were all dried up (forever). Should you like to coopt this masterpiece:

> Being patient,
> Being patient,
> It's so hard!
> It's so hard!
> But it's so important,
> Yes, it's so important.
> So we try.
> So we try.

Now, whenever my kids start to lose their patience, I look them in the eye and start singing this song. More often than not, they join in, and we sing together until I can meet their needs.

👍 DO be willing to look silly.

Toddlers love silly, especially when it comes from all-business Mom or buttoned-up Dad. As I said, surprise can be your friend. Worried about how you'll look bursting into (off-key) song in the middle of the big-box store? Embarrassed to challenge your three-year-old to a jumping race down the path out of the playground so as to make the necessary exit? Expanding your repertoire of tantrum prevention and deescalation strategies can feel like learning a new instrument, sport, or language, and you may not feel comfortable displaying your amateur status in public. Trust me, though, and try out new strategies even if you think you'll look dumb; I'd bet it'll turn out to be worth the risk.

👍 DO develop an awareness of your own states.

When your two-year-old is clearly descending into yet another emotional collapse, you may feel you're all too aware of your current state of aggravation, exhaustion, and despair. But often it's important to be aware of how you're feeling—emotionally, mentally, and physically—even before you see signs of an oncoming storm, because it's your compromised condition that may very well be causing the clouds to gather. Know when you're stressed—rushed and tired in the grocery store, starving due to having been too busy at work to eat before you picked up your preschooler, distracted and worried about a relative or friend. Toddlers have finely tuned senses for parents' stress, and your tension can make them feel they've lost some of the support they usually count on to handle their own emotions. I'm not suggesting that you remain supernaturally calm and cheery at all times; that wouldn't fit at all with the push for authenticity I've been making in the preceding chapters. You just need to foster an awareness of these states so that you can be extra prepared and take the appropriate measures (laid out in this and the next three chapters) to head off a tantrum.

These three strategies—and more—are based on an understanding of your role in the tantrum dance with your toddler or preschooler, offered in Chapter 4. If you haven't read it yet, consider doing so, particularly if you ever start wondering how a grown-up can repeatedly be outmatched by a two-and-a-half-year-old.

Know Who You're Dealing With

I noted in Chapter 2 that I've met parents who have actually asked me (more than once) if I was sure their three-foot-tall child wasn't a psychopath. If you've felt bested far too often by your three-and-a-half-year-old, you might be pondering the same question. No, your little guy is not severely disturbed; he's just, well, a little guy. It's important to know where kids this young are limited because of their developmental stage—and to respond accordingly. Here are some key strategies.

🔒 DO see the world from your toddler or preschooler's perspective.

I recently did a consultation for a family with two children, Maddie and Aidan, ages two and a half and four. Part of the consultation included an observation of the family during a "typical" time at home, in this case dinner followed by the transition to the bath. Once the children were in the tub, the nanny took over, and I met with their parents, Mike and Sherri, to provide feedback. Sherri suggested we meet in her home office, which was down the hall from the bathroom where Maddie and Aidan were wrapping up their baths, and the bedrooms where they would soon be going to sleep.

A few minutes after we began our conversation, there was a knock on the door. "What you doing?" Maddie asked innocently. Mike responded that we were in a meeting for grown-ups and that we'd be done soon. This response, while harmless on its face, was going to be problematic for two reasons. First, two-year-olds notoriously hate being made aware that they are not grown-ups, or—even more generally—that they are not welcome where others are. Second, it was patently untrue that we were going to be done soon; we had just begun. "Stop having a meeting for grown-ups," Maddie demanded. "I no like that!" Soon Aidan was standing behind his sister: "Mom, can I have some milk?" Sherri let out an audible exhale. "Aidan, Mommy and Daddy are busy right now." Within a few minutes of this, both kids were in full-on meltdown mode and Sherri and Mike weren't far behind. We ended up rescheduling the feedback session for the following week.

During that subsequent session, the first question Sherri asked was how to respond when Maddie gets "bossy" with them, such as when she demanded that they stop our meeting. To their minds, this was where and how the tantrum began. I offer strategies later in this chapter that Mike and Sherri might have used to head off Maddie's tantrum, but I wanted to start way before that, because so much of preventing and managing tantrums involves what happened earlier. Why, I asked, out of all the rooms on all three floors, had they chosen Sherri's home office as the room in which to hold the feedback session? Mike responded first: "It seemed like the most comfortable room to have a conversation like that." Then Sherri: "And we were all already right there; we didn't need to go downstairs or anything." Then it was my turn: "What would have happened, do you think, if we'd chosen to meet in the dining room, or even the basement?" My point was that the entire situation—the whining, crying, yelling, falling on the floor—could most likely have been avoided if Sherri and Mike had made the decision of where to hold the meeting with *their children's viewpoints*, rather than their own preferences, primary in their minds. Which leads me to the next key strategy.

👍 DO think ahead.

If Sherri and Mike had thought ahead about how their choice of meeting place might affect their children, things might have turned out differently. Sometimes when I have this conversation with parents, suggesting that they think about their children's perspective and anticipate what might happen, they respond in a puzzled manner; after all, what parents aren't thinking about their child's feelings and needs 24/7? The key, though, is that an important part of tantrum prevention involves not only thinking about your toddler's needs but also actually seeing the world through your child's eyes. That power—of perspective taking, or reflective functioning (defined as the capacity to imagine both one's own and others' mental states)—is undoubtedly one of the most potent in your repertoire. (There is a vast body of research about the relationship between reflective functioning and positive child outcomes.)

A few weeks ago, I picked up some dried mango as a treat for Henry while he was at preschool, then came home and offhandedly put the bag on the kitchen counter. A couple of hours later, Henry came into the kitchen to have dinner, at which point his eyes landed on the mango with a laserlike focus. "I want mango!" he demanded. And, just like that, I had an impending tantrum to attempt to derail.

Let me be clear: this looming meltdown was unequivocally my own fault. Had I remembered that, at Henry's height, the counter is exactly at eye level, I would have thought to put the dried mango in the pantry with the other snacks. Henry would not have seen it right before dinner, would not have asked for it, would not have been told no, and would not have started to lose his mind. It's like a game of dominoes, with parents having the power to place the first domino where it won't knock down any others if it falls. This makes for a very unexciting and unimpressive domino chain, of course, but it happens to be exactly what you want when it comes to a tantrum. I once saw a client who complained that her son was always drawing with permanent markers, no matter how many times she told him not to. "There are marker stains on everything!" she exclaimed. It turns out she kept the markers in a holder on the wall that her son *could reach*. I suggested she keep the markers somewhere else. I got paid for that. (OK, OK, I made a few other suggestions as well.) Taking your little one's perspective means being aware of the space she inhabits, the times of day that are hardest, the things he loves, the things she hates. . . .

> Parents have the power to stop the domino effect that leads to a tantrum by placing the first domino where it won't knock over the next.

"But I can't always think that far ahead!" a father said to me recently. "It's exhausting!" Yes, it is. At first. As are sit-ups when you've never done them before. But they get easier with time and practice. And no, you won't "always" be able to think that far ahead— let's avoid impossible parenting standards, people—but you'll be able to do so more and more, and every little bit will help.

👍 *DO help your child develop emotional fluency from an early age.*

See the *do* on page 155 regarding labeling and reflecting your child's emotions when he is starting to get frustrated and a tantrum is on the near horizon. When toddlers have a tantrum because they can't manage emotional distress, it often starts with not even knowing what emotion they are experiencing. Learning names for feelings and how to express emotional states using words can reduce the frequency of tantrums and is also critical for optimizing social emotional development. You can build this learning into your daily interactions with your toddler or preschooler. Various children's books have been written expressly for this purpose, many of which are quite fun to read with your child (see the Resources).

Remember That All of Us Do as People Do, Not as They Say

I have a confession. When Zeke was an infant, sometimes I picked his nose (look, he was a winter baby, I wanted him to be able to breathe, and that suction bulb thingy is worthless). Several months ago Zeke started crying, and when I turned around, I saw that Henry was picking his (that is, Zeke's) nose—just going all up in there. Although I certainly never intended to model picking Zeke's nose, I had apparently done so, and quite effectively. The lesson:

👍 DO think about what you do—because you'll see your child mimic it.

Toddlers and preschoolers are watching your every move. They "talk on the phone," "go to the supermarket," and say they'll be there "in two minutes." Sometimes we learn this the hard way: they use a curse word we didn't realize they'd overheard, or draw a picture of a glass of red wine and ask it to be titled "Mommy's favorite" (this happened to a friend of mine). Like it or not, parents are their children's nonstop role models.

The problem is that we—parents, and adults in general—are very good at saying one thing and doing another. In 2016–2017, I served as the director of early childhood programming for an amazing nonprofit organization called Ramapo for Children, which has a very effective way of demonstrating this principle. Specifically, as an experiential exercise, a facilitator explains that she will say "1, 2, 3, go" and that participants—generally a group of adults who work with children in some capacity—will clap on the word "go." The facilitator repeats the instructions and checks for understanding until everyone is clear. The facilitator then says "1, 2, 3, go" as planned, except instead of clapping on "go," the facilitator herself claps on "3." At which point most of the participants—all of whom are looking at the facilitator—also clap on three, with only a few waiting until "go" to clap, as instructed. Why does this happen? *Because, in contrast to the popular adage, human beings tend to do as people do, not as they say.*

 DO pay particular attention to modeling healthy emotion regulation.

When it comes to tantrums, the most important thing we model is how we handle our emotions. Ask yourself: What do you look like when you're angry or upset? Do you curse like a sailor when someone cuts you off on the highway or when your computer freezes? Slam your bedroom door when you feel disappointed or let down? Once you have a child, these behaviors—like everything else—are not only about you. How your child learns to handle his or her difficult feelings is going to depend a great deal on how she sees you handling yours (of course, there's also the genetic/temperamental component to emotional reactivity, as discussed in Chapter 5). If you, like the father described in Chapter 4, start to take three deep breaths when you feel frustrated—and to say out loud that this is what you're doing—your child may well learn to do that too. If you talk about taking a break when you're angry (for example, "Wow—I really feel like throwing the pieces of this desk across the room instead of putting it together; it's clearly time for me to stop for a little while"), that's a skill your child will adopt.

> Regulating your emotions is one of the most important things you can model for a toddler or preschooler.

One time I was doing an in-home observation for parents whose four-year-old son, Haran, was having frequent tantrums at his preschool. He had recently thrown a box of crayons after "messing up" his drawing and had kicked a classmate after he was unable to learn the clapping motions to a song. I was already in the family's home when Haran's father returned from work and went upstairs to change. After a few moments, a yell came from the upstairs bedroom: "F*&%!" Haran's mother looked concerned; "What is it, honey?" she yelled up the stairs. More yelling: "I left the shirts on the train! I don't believe this! I am such an idiot!" It seems that Haran's father had spent his lunch hour buying himself a couple of new shirts and then accidentally left them on the train during his evening commute. The father's self-flagellation didn't end there; for the next 20 minutes, he shook his head and berated himself out loud for his error.

A couple of quick points. First, this family was, by pretty much any standard, quite wealthy. Even the wealthiest of us, of course, don't like to throw money away, but it's important to know that losing a couple of new shirts was not going to result in any financial hardship. Second, I am not suggesting that Haran's tantrums were solely the result of his emulating his father's frustration around making mistakes. As is most often the case, Haran's tantrums were triggered by numerous factors that were undoubtedly operating along more than one pathway (see Chapter 2). It was clear in that moment, however, that Haran's father's difficulty with tolerating frustration was likely contributing to Haran's disruptive behavior in preschool. In other words, Haran's father was modeling the very behavior that he wanted his son to stop.

In our subsequent work together, Haran's father became aware of the extent to which adjusting his own behavior might, in turn, decrease his son's tantrums in school. A few months later, Haran's father noticed a ticket for an expired inspection on his windshield. "All I wanted to do," he told me, "was slam my head into the steering wheel; I couldn't believe that I'd let the inspection lapse without even noticing!" But he didn't: "I remembered that Haran was in the backseat and that he was watching me. I turned around and told him I felt frustrated about a mistake I'd made and that I needed to take three deep breaths before we could drive home. Actually, Haran then counted for me while I smelled the flowers and blew out the candles [this is a great way to teach deep breathing to young kids—inhale as if smelling a flower, exhale as if blowing out birthday candles]—it was pretty funny." In this case, Haran's father's work on his own behavior led not only to a decrease in Haran's tantrums, but also to a closer and more connected father–son relationship, which, remember, is foundational in all of this (see Chapter 6).

👍 DO apologize.

One additional area in which modeling plays a key role is that of the *apology*. Parents frequently resist apologizing to their little ones when they lose their cool. Some parents feel as though they shouldn't *have* to apologize for their behavior, that to do so is somehow placing their child in a position of power. Others assume that an apology will call too much attention to an occurrence that they would rather brush under the rug. The thing is, toddlers and preschoolers are human, and so are parents. Humans make mistakes, and when they do, it's generally considered appropriate—as well as kind and considerate—to apologize. If you would like, over time, to teach your child to apologize when he loses control of his temper, then much more effective than the conventional (and, to my mind, way overused and often ineffective) "say you're sorry" approach is to model this behavior yourself.

> Demonstrate the power of the apology to your toddler by saying you're sorry when you lose control of your temper.

A little over a year ago, I snapped at Henry when he cheerily marched into Zeke's room and began singing at the top of his lungs just as I was laying Zeke—asleep at last—in his crib. "I do *not* want you in here!" I still remember hissing, daggers shooting out of my eyes, "You get out of here *now!*" Henry left the room, only to collapse into a mess of tears in the hallway. After Zeke was (finally) sleeping, I approached him; he'd stopped crying but still looked pretty upset. He looked up at me. "Mommy no want me Zekey's room?" "No," I responded. "It was time for Zekey to go to sleep, and I was afraid that your very loud singing was going to wake him up." "Oh. (*Long pause.*) Mommy want I go away?" All I wanted to say was *no,* of course not, that I'd *never* want him to go away! I love him to pieces! And let's go play a fun game! And forget the whole thing ever happened! La la la la la! But I didn't. I knew I'd lost my temper and needed to acknowledge and apologize for that. Why? Because I feel strongly that these are important skills for him to develop as he gets older. "I did want you to go away in that moment," I explained. "Because I was angry, and afraid you were going to wake up your brother. I am sorry I spoke to you in a mean tone of voice." Henry nodded. "I need you to work on being quiet when Zeke is sleeping," I continued, because this was still very much true—this limit was important. "And I'm sorry for losing my temper." Because that part, although harder to say out loud, was also very much true.

Apologizing is one way to repair after a rupture in the all-important authentic connection between you and your toddler, a concept introduced in Chapter 6 and discussed later in this book as well.

 DO *model the specific behaviors you want to see from your toddler.*

The bottom line about modeling is quite simple—certainly to say, if not to do (fitting, right?). As much as possible, parents need to demonstrate the behaviors that they would like their toddlers to demonstrate. Even if you enact every single other strategy perfectly, if you yourself (or another parent or frequent caregiver) are having difficulty handling big emotions, then you will likely be unable to handle your child's tantrums in an effective manner.

Chapter 4 is worth reviewing if you want to think more about your specific emotion regulation capabilities.

Using Attention Wisely

I have discussed the idea of paying "strategic attention" with countless families, and I am almost always met with the same comment: "Attention? Oh come *on*. This child already gets so much attention, you don't even know. Trust me: attention is not the problem." And so I highlight that first word: *strategic*. This strategy is about using your attention as a *tool*, being smart about it, understanding the power it holds, and choosing to harness it for good. It's not simply about giving your toddler or preschooler *more* attention, but about learning *how* to give attention in a way that leads to fewer tantrums and improved behavior more generally.

We, as human beings, are all motivated by the possibility of a reward, expected or otherwise. When we are rewarded for a particular behavior, we tend to do it again and again; the reward reinforces the behavior. Yesterday, I went to a deli to grab lunch; when I went to pay, the cashier pushed my hand back. "It's on me," he said with a smile. "Thanks for being so happy and energetic today." I will clearly be going back there for lunch and will do my best to bring out my happiest and most energetic. (For what it's worth, what the cashier called "energetic" I would call "completely amped up on caffeine due to my child's sleep strike the night before," but whatever. Details.)

 DO use your attention as a reward for behavior you want to encourage.

Toddlers and preschoolers are no different. So what is the number-one reward for young children, the thing they want more than anything else in the whole world? The answer is YOU: their parents. More than anything else in the whole world, toddlers and preschoolers want attention from their parents. And so it follows logically that whatever behaviors get the most attention from their parents are the behaviors that young children are going to repeat again and again. And again. And again.

This principle plays out all the time during the winter, when kids refuse to put on their jackets, despite the cold temperatures. I worked with one such three-year-old, Lily, and her mother, Helen. Helen described getting out of the house as "agonizing," as Lily would "throw a fit" every time she needed to put on her jacket. One morning I observed as Helen packed for a morning at music class, checking (and double-checking) that she had in her bag diapers, wipes, snacks, her wallet, her phone, a sippy cup, her lipstick, her keys, hand sanitizer, a change of clothes for Lily, her own gloves, Lily's mittens, her own hat, Lily's hat, Lily's lovey, a pack of gum . . . Finally, it was time for Lily to put on her shoes and her jacket. "Come here, Lily," Helen said. "It's time to put your shoes on." Lily walked over to her mom, who bent down and put her shoes on Lily's feet while Lily held on to her shoulder. Helen then stood up and turned around to get Lily's jacket. "And now your jacket," she said. As if on cue, Lily took the opportunity to run to the other side of the room. "*Now,*" Helen said. "No," Lily responded. "I said *now,*" from Mom. "No" from Lily.

Things devolved quickly from there. Lily was soon a flailing, tantruming mess, and Helen was pleading with her to pull it together so that they could go to music class—"which you love!" I don't remember exactly how Helen finally managed to get Lily to put her jacket on, but it took at least 10 minutes, and there was a cookie involved.

> If your toddler gets your attention by throwing a tantrum, how likely is he to use this strategy?

Are toddlers impervious to cold by nature? Is there some unspoken toddler understanding that to don one's jacket is a sign of weakness? No to both. The fact is, toddlers typically get a ton more attention for refusing to put on their jackets than for putting them on as instructed. When Helen asked Lily to come put her shoes on, Lily did so; she walked directly over to her mother and allowed her shoes to be put on her feet without protest. That piece of the interaction—let's call it part one—took all of about one minute. And how did Helen respond? She turned her back to Lily and asked her to do something else (put on her jacket). Now, if you're a toddler who values attention from Mom more than anything else, have you been rewarded for this exchange? No. Compare it, though, with part two, in which Lily refuses to put on her jacket and ends up getting ten extra minutes of Mom time. Rewarding? Yes. In short: When young children put on their jackets right away, parents *may* say "thank you" or "good job," but that's generally about it. When young children don't put on their jackets right away, they get several extra minutes of time with a parent, during which the attention is solely on them. In their world, this is called *hitting the jackpot*. When I gave Helen this feedback, she looked incredulous. "But I don't understand; Lily *loves* music class. And she gets so much of my attention there! If she's rewarded by my attention, why wouldn't she want to get there as soon as possible?"

To answer Helen's question, we have to refer back to the first strategy mentioned and see the situation from *Lily's* perspective:

1. As we know from Chapter 3, toddlers and preschoolers live in the moment; their brains are not able to plan ahead. If they are getting attention in the present moment, that supersedes all.

2. Unlike adults, toddlers and preschoolers often prefer negative attention to no attention. So, for example, if I, an adult, have a choice between my best friend's being too busy to check in with me for a few weeks or her reaching out to express how angry and upset she is with me, I'll undoubtedly opt for the former. Young children are the opposite. For them, any attention is better than no attention at all, which is why refusing to put on a jacket typically beats putting on a jacket at the first request. As a general rule, toddlers and preschoolers will choose attention over no attention, even if this attention comes in the form of chastising or scolding.

Once Helen understood these two points, she started to see results. She began to pay more attention to Lily when she *did* put on her shoes or jacket right away and less attention when she did not. The battles around getting out of the house decreased in frequency and duration, and both Helen and Lily could enjoy music class (and wherever else they were headed).

Strategic attention, then, means purposefully giving more attention to a behavior you want to promote (such as following directions) than to a behavior you want to eliminate (defiance, for example), with the goal of increasing the former and decreasing the latter.

 DO pull out your phone when your child is starting to melt down, not when he's behaving calmly.

Strategic attention can also be as simple as choosing when to be present and focused on your child and when not to be. Think: smartphones. We always take out our phones when our children are playing nicely by themselves, eating quietly, or generally engaging in behavior that we want. "Sweet," we think to ourselves, consciously or not. "I can return that email I've had flagged since this morning." Sure enough, the moment we take out our phone, our little one smushes an Oreo into the couch or pitches a block at the wall. At that point we put our phones away to chastise the behavior, and—voilà!—we have once again rewarded the behavior we *don't* want rather than the one we *do*.

> Calmly ignoring behavior that you want to discourage can be as effective as paying attention to behavior you want to encourage.

If we follow the principle of strategic attention, we don't want to use our phones when our toddlers and preschoolers are engaged in desirable behaviors. But when they begin to engage in undesirable behaviors—like, say, the beginning of a tantrum—phone time! *Because the opposite of attending to a behavior is ignoring it,* and sometimes if you ignore the behaviors that signal an oncoming tantrum (feet stomping, grunting), your toddler will get the message and cease and desist.

 DO use cheerleading—even (and maybe even especially) for small victories.

In her work with parents, a former colleague (and longtime friend), Dr. Lesli Preuss, refers to certain types of strategic attention as cheerleading, which I've found to be a very helpful analogy. It can feel strange to give your child attention for tolerating frustration as opposed to having a meltdown or for following directions instead of staging a full-on protest. Kids should *know* that these behaviors are preferable, we argue, and therefore just *do* them; why do we need to make a big deal about it when they're just doing what they're supposed to be doing? First, as you saw in Chapter 3, just because young children know something doesn't mean they can necessarily act on it; impulsivity reigns in this age group. Second, this stuff works.

Professional athletes know what's expected of them; they are being paid to hit a home run, score a touchdown, or make a basket. Does this mean we don't cheer them on because they already know what to do and what we, their fans, will appreciate? Do we say, "Well, he's on third and knows his job is to run home, so no need for me to get involved"? No! We cheer like crazy. We cheer because our cheering—and the implied support and encouragement behind it—*helps*. At the end of a really hard day—the kind when you and your child have been butting heads since the moment she woke up—the last thing in the world you feel like doing is highlighting the positive in your child. Parents will look at me incredulously: "He's been screaming and crying all day, and now you want me to be happy because he managed to keep himself together just once?" Yes. Why? *Because the hardest days are the ones on which he'll need it most.* If our team finally scores for the first time at the bottom of the eighth inning, do we stay quiet? Do we roll our eyes and let them know that it's a little late to step up their performance? Nope. Again: we cheer like crazy. Because they are down and out, and because knowing we're on their side—rooting for them 100% from the sidelines—may be just what they need to turn the game around.

Right before the Tantrum: Catch That Train Before It Runs Off the Track

If you use the preceding strategies on most days, there's a pretty good chance that your toddler's tantrums will become fewer and farther between. But there are times when you can see a tantrum coming, like an oncoming train (do I need to repeat the fact that tantrums are normal?), and need more tools to head it off.

Give Your Child Credit

Sometimes when parents tell me their child's tantrums seem to come out of the blue and they're becoming more frequent, I have to ask them to review with me what has happened before several of these eruptions—right before, within a few hours of the tantrum, or even for the whole day. They often tell me stories like this one:

Over the phone, two-and-a-half-year-old Dante's parents had shared with me that he was having tantrums over "every little thing" that didn't go his way. Upon observation, I saw Dante (1) be told that he could not have another cheese stick, (2) watch his baby brother accidentally knock down a block tower he was building, and (3) have to wait until his mother stopped texting for her to answer his question about dinosaurs. In the wake of each of these three incidents—incidents I expected to end in tantrums, based on his parents' account—Dante remained calm. Right before I was leaving, however, Dante asked his father if he could read one more book before bath time. When Dante's father said no, Dante threw himself down on the ground in despair, prompting his father to look at me with a "You see?" expression. Dante's father then spent approximately five minutes attempting to appease Dante, ultimately acquiescing and reading one more book.

What was happening here? The explanation was plain, and so was the solution:

DO remain aware of all the frustrations your child has handled effectively.

Dante got absolutely zero attention for handling frustration in the way his parents wanted him to, by staying calm; in fact, it almost seemed as though his parents didn't notice all of the occasions on which he was able to demonstrate impressive coping skills. Conversely, the one time Dante was not able to handle his frustration well and a tantrum ensued, his father gave him more, and more intensive, attention than he had gotten all evening. Dante was slowly learning that tantrums = more attention, and so the episodes were becoming more frequent. And so what would the use of strategic attention by Dante's parents look like in this scenario?

 DO pay strategic attention to your child's successes.

The goal, remember, is to draw attention to those behaviors you want to promote, in this case Dante's capacity for staying calm, for regulating his emotions even when faced with potentially frustrating circumstances: "Wow! Look how you stayed calm when Mommy told you no more cheese sticks; you really are learning how to handle getting an answer you don't like!" When making these comments, it can be helpful to focus on your child's agency: "You just made a choice to stay calm even though your brother knocked down your tower; you're really learning how much power you have!"

Zero In on Your Toddler's Emotions

A few months ago I was running late to see a client. I called my husband during my speed-walk to her building and recounted the morning's pitfalls, including an epic traffic jam and lack of parking. Unlike when I checked in with him about the fender bender (see Chapter 6), this time, no doubt with the best of intentions, he made a suggestion: "You know, you should probably leave earlier, give yourself more of a cushion." I felt my muscles tighten and my heart pound faster. "That's not the point," I snapped before reiterating, more loudly and forcefully, the saga of my morning commute. In other words, I started to have a tantrum. All I wanted in that moment was to be "gotten," that is, heard and understood. It was not the time for logic, and I wasn't in the mood for tips on self-improvement. It's not that my husband was wrong; quite the opposite, in fact. But I was already upset, and all I wanted to hear was "Honey, that sounds awful," or even just, as in the case of the fender bender, an understanding "Ugh."

 DO skip the rational explanation.

Too often, when toddlers and preschoolers are on the verge of tantrums, we intervene with logic, with rational explanations or arguments intended to decrease frustration. And yet in doing so—with the best of intentions— we make things worse. Our child's initial frustration becomes compounded because she feels neither heard nor understood. A mother I saw recently, Nancy, had forgotten to get more milk for her family after they ran out one morning. That evening, her two-year-old, Caryn, staged a protest: "I want milk!" she yelled over and over again. Each time, Nancy responded by explaining that there *was* no milk. This response only agitated Caryn further, which of course led Nancy to become frustrated as well. Here, Caryn's tantrum started because she wanted and couldn't get milk, but then intensified because her mother simply didn't seem to understand how upsetting this was. Caryn was not asking whether there was more milk—she may well have understood, especially after the third time she was told, that there was none on hand. Rather, she was saying she wanted some; regardless of the objective reality of the situation, she wanted milk and she wanted milk *now*.

 DO label and reflect your child's emotions when a tantrum seems imminent.

What Nancy needed to do in that moment was to acknowledge Caryn's desire and frustration by describing what was going on: "I know, sweetie. I get it. You *really, really* want milk, and I'm saying you can't have any."

In some ways, approaching an impending tantrum by labeling and reflecting feelings is counterintuitive. Our instinct as parents is frequently to "fix it" when children feel angry or frustrated, in part to avoid the dreaded meltdown, and in part because no one enjoys seeing his or her child upset. The problem, however, is that when we do this, we run the risk of not meeting our children where they are, of neglecting to empathize with their emotional experiences. This, in turn, actually *increases* the likelihood that a tantrum will occur or intensify. After all, when you communicate to your child that you genuinely don't understand how upset she is or why, how will she respond? By trying to *get* you to understand, to *make* you understand, which means crying more, yelling louder, and stomping her feet harder.

I worked with a father, Ryan, who, due to his work schedule, was never able to drop his son off at day care in the mornings. He and his wife contacted me because their son was having a huge tantrum each morning. "Daddy, I want *you* to take me, not Mommy," he would whine, then cry, scream, kick, and so forth. Every time this happened Ryan would inform his son how lucky he was that his mother was the one to take him to day care. "Mom's much more fun than I am in the mornings," he would say. "I'm so boring and tired. Trust me; Mom is definitely the best person for the job!" Ryan was trying so hard to make his son feel better (and likely to alleviate his own guilt), and yet his efforts had the opposite effect. I recommended that Ryan try something new, that he empathize with where his son was coming from. He was skeptical but reported a week later that this strategy had worked, that his son was no longer having tantrums in the morning. What were the magic words? I don't remember them exactly, but something along the lines of "I know, buddy; I so wish I could take you. It really stinks that I have to go to work instead." Boom. Two sentences. No more morning tantrums.

👍 DO keep it short.

Here, the brevity piece—Ryan's response was a mere two sentences—is important, lest this strategy come into conflict with that of "strategic attention." You don't want to give your child so much empathy leading up to a tantrum that the reflection of emotions becomes a way of rewarding the behavior you want to decrease. Had Ryan sat down with his son for 20 minutes to talk about how he wished he could take him to day care, the daily tantrums may not have subsided so quickly (although talking about this at another time would certainly be OK). It doesn't take much, though; sometimes simply reflecting back how your child is feeling is enough for her to feel heard, and thus to calm down. Becoming comfortable saying things like "Wow, you seem so frustrated right now" or "I can see how much you want to watch another show" is essential for stopping tantrums before they reach their boiling point. The goal is to connect—to communicate that you get it and are on the same team—and then to back off, providing the space for your child to feel the emotions he feels. Not the ones you *think* he should feel, but the ones he *does* feel.

> When you see resistance brewing in your toddler, skip the rational argument and try reflecting and labeling the child's emotions.

See Chapter 6: If tantrums are a manifestation of overwhelming emotions, then knowing you are present and supportive does much to decrease the overwhelm (and, therefore, the tantrum itself).

A couple more quick *dos* on this strategy:

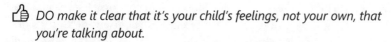 **DO make it clear that it's your child's feelings, not your own, that you're talking about.**

You'll notice in the examples on the previous pages that labeling feelings is actually, more precisely, checking in about feelings. Using words like "seem" or inserting a "huh" at the end of an assumption about what your child is experiencing simultaneously offers guidance and communicates that the experience is *his, not yours,* thereby delineating an important boundary between parent and child. The idea is to help little ones learn to recognize and feel comfortable with their own feelings, not for us to tell them how they should or do feel. Communicating the latter, even unintentionally, runs the risk that they will learn to look to others in the future to decode their feelings, rather than to do so on their own. Another effective way to handle this issue is to describe the facts of a situation—essentially to narrate it, sportscaster style—without using any emotion words at all. For example, "I see that you were playing with the farm animals, and then Mark came over and took the cow out of the barn without asking, and now you're crying." Of course, if you go this route, you need to make sure that you're speaking in an empathic tone, or else you run the risk of sounding a bit robotic, which will not have the desired calming effect.

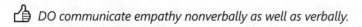 **DO communicate empathy nonverbally as well as verbally.**

Although "labeling" and "describing" imply the use of verbal communication, it's important to note that one's affect, facial expression, and body language are also ways to communicate empathy. If you do use words, their meaning needs to be congruent with these other modes of communication for this strategy to have an impact. Your child needs to know you genuinely mean it when you express empathy for her feelings if you are to stave off a tantrum.

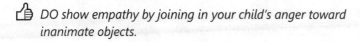 **DO show empathy by joining in your child's anger toward inanimate objects.**

I recently met with a mother whose daughter, Kaya, kept having tantrums when playing with her favorite doll. Although Kaya constantly wanted to change the doll's clothes, she didn't yet have the fine motor coordination to be able to do so, and she would end up throwing the clothes across the room in a fit of frustration. Her mother had tried helping Kaya by showing her how to put the clothes on the doll and had also attempted to be empathic about how disappointing it can be not to be able to do something well at first. When these approaches didn't seem to work, I suggested she join in her daughter's irritation with the clothes themselves. "But it's not really the clothes' fault," this mother said. "Of course it is!" I responded. To illustrate the approach, I continued: "Stupid clothes! Get on my doll already! Why can't you just get on easier? You are the worst clothes in the whole wide world!" My thought was that if Mom could express these kinds of sentiments, she would be (1) adding some humor/levity to the situation, (2) putting words to and thereby validating her daughter's emotional experience, and (3) connecting with her daughter by being on the same team. Not a bad trifecta for managing a tantrum, right? After all, it wasn't like we needed to worry about the *clothes'* feelings.

Tap the Power of Distraction

Distraction is a deceptively simple way to avert a tantrum. It involves shifting your child's focus using the old "Ooh, look over there!" or "Here's something shiny!" trick. At first glance it may seem as though this strategy is in direct conflict with that of labeling and reflecting emotions. After all, we just emphasized the importance of acknowledging and appreciating your child's feelings. Remember, these strategies are best when mixed and matched and blended seamlessly; different ones are more and less effective for different children and in different situations. You don't want to distract your child every time he is upset about something, as you'll run the risk of invalidating his emotional experience, which will take a substantive toll on your relationship (see Chapter 6). That said, it's also OK to follow a comment that labels your child's emotion ("You seem really frustrated") with a distracting joke, story, or song. This is a particularly useful technique when you can almost see a tantrum taking shape, say when your child is tired, or hungry, or just found out he can't have ice cream after dinner and seems to be pondering his next move . . .

 DO ask a question that seems to come out of the blue.

One of my favorites is "Hey, do you remember what you had for breakfast this morning [or, if it's morning, dinner last night]?" Most kids won't be able to recall this right away (if at all), and their subsequent pause will serve the dual purpose of taking their mind off their distress and buying you time to think about where you're going to take the conversation. And then it's just about thinking on your feet. Let's say your child pauses and then remembers that he had scrambled eggs for breakfast. You could:

- Tell him about how eggs come from chickens.
- Go into the age-old puzzling question of what came first, the chicken or the egg.
- Have a contest to see how many different kinds of eggs he can name (scrambled, hard-boiled, omelet, etc.). This will, of course, work only in big egg-eating families. We happen to be one.
- Ask what color scrambled eggs are and what other things (in general, or in the room) are yellow.
- Make up a song about eggs ("Old McDonald had some eggs, E-I-E-I-O, and on his eggs he had some salt, E-I-E-I-O . . ." Just made that up right now. I swear. You can thank me later.)
- Ask what letter "egg" starts with and think of other things that start with "E."
- Say what a funny word "scrambled" is, then just start making up funny-sounding words and speaking nonsense language.
- Ask what rhymes with "egg."
- Ask him whether Elmo/Buzz Lightyear/Elsa/Minions/Chase/Rocky/Moana/Trolls like eggs, and how, and with what, and so forth.
- See who can say "scrambled eggs" the quietest.

You now have 10 ways to distract your child from a possible tantrum using only the information that he had scrambled eggs for breakfast. The key is to be creative and run with whatever information you have in the moment.

> Distraction is endlessly powerful in heading off a tantrum, but don't use it endlessly, or you risk invalidating your toddler's emotional experience.

 DO *challenge your child to a race.*

When in doubt, have a race. Young kids love racing, especially racing against *you*, and you should take advantage of this as much as possible. Impending tantrum about not wanting to take a bath? Race to the tub. Meltdown on the horizon about not wanting to sit down for dinner? Use a stopwatch to see how fast she can get to the table and in her seat. On the brink of falling apart due to desire for candy at the supermarket? Race to see who can spot the broccoli first. And remember, races come in all shapes and sizes. Choose your base ingredient: running, jumping, crawling, or spinning, m*aybe* hopping if your child is extra coordinated. Then add your topping: with your hands on your head, while oinking like a pig, while singing "Twinkle, Twinkle," without moving your arms, etcetera.

 DO challenge the toddler/preschooler to do something all by herself.

Three other magic words that go under the distraction heading: *all by your-self.* As in "I bet you can't do [insert whatever you can think of here] all by yourself!" This may relate to the tantrum-inducing task itself, as in "I bet you can't get undressed for your bath all by yourself!" Or you might use this strategy completely out of left field, as in the following exchange:

CALEB: I want a lollipop!

MOM: I know you do, honey. Lollipops are delicious. Hey, I bet you can't stand on one foot all by yourself!

Sounds crazy, right? But toddlers and preschoolers eat it up; remember, at this stage of their development they are craving opportunities to demonstrate their autonomy (see Chapter 3). In this example, though, the "I know you do, honey" part and the acknowledgment that lollipops are delicious are important components too. If you skip right to the standing-on-one-foot contest without noting that you hear the lollipop request, you might just get a louder request, and then a louder request, and then a screaming request, and then a screaming and crying request . . .

Honestly, I could write 100 pages on this strategy alone, because there are always more possible ways to distract young children; it's just a matter of choosing your favorites, which means the ones that come most easily to you and are most effective for your particular child. Three more top picks:

 DO have your child be a "helper."

Toddlers and preschoolers love "helping" (quotation marks to indicate that it is the perception of helping and not whether their help is actually valuable that is important here). Ask your child to help you unload groceries, wipe the table, fold laundry, bring this piece of paper to Mommy, check to see if the car is still outside, tell you how many pillows are on the couch, and so on. Preface with "Can you please be super helpful and . . . ?" The only caveat is that if you are using this technique as a means of distraction, do not then inadvertently step into a power struggle trap or an opportunity to criticize your child. If he says, "No! I won't!" then let it be, rather than argue or point out how "not nice" he is being. It's a strategy aimed at making things better, not worse. If it yields the latter, time to drop it.

DO introduce a prop.

Yes, once in a while this can be your phone; desperate times sometimes call for desperate measures. I'd limit phone use (as a distraction technique, not with regard to screen time more generally, which is a different topic) to exactly that, though—desperate times. Your phone is a reward, by definition, in that it's shiny and colorful and interesting and fancy and delicate. You don't want to start rewarding your child's about-to-have-a-tantrum signs with use of the phone. Also, once you begin to rely on your phone, other props—a book, a toy, a spoon, a straw—stop working, and then you've dug yourself into a bit of a hole.

DO imitate your child.

Imitate, don't mock. If you are actively feeling angry at your child (go back to Chapter 4 and read about how important it is to be aware of your own triggers/emotions), this is not a great technique to use, as it runs the risk of becoming mean-spirited ridicule. If you can genuinely find humor in a situation, however—the loving, connected kind—then this can be a wonderful tool to have at your disposal. If your child says, "No, don't change my diaper!" you simply respond, "No, you don't change MY diaper!" Or follow "Pick me up! Pick me up now!" with "No, you pick ME up! Pick ME up now!" I can almost guarantee that your toddler will pause, look puzzled, and maybe even smile. And once there's a smile—or even a puzzled pause—you're golden, well on your way to "Whew, I think we successfully avoided tantrum town."

Offer Choices

Sometimes, as parents, it feels like our little ones have the best lives in the world. And in many ways they do. They are 100% taken care of, always, never having to worry about when or what they're going to eat, paying the bills, current affairs, or politics. The flip side of this, though, is that they have almost no autonomy. They are told what to eat, when to eat, and where to eat; they are told when and where to sleep; they are told what to wear, how to spend their days, and who to spend them with. This is all happening, as we discussed in Chapter 3, at the exact same time that, from a developmental perspective, toddlers and preschoolers are craving independence, learning to assert control over their environment, and experimenting with what circumstances they can and cannot dictate. Giving choices is a strategy that provides children with a sense of agency, thereby helping to alleviate the tension that arises between the reality—that they can't control the vast majority of their experiences or environments—and the yearning for autonomy that they feel. Take breakfast time. You might ask your child whether she wants eggs or a waffle, as well as her preferred chair at the table.

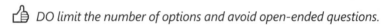 *DO limit the number of options and avoid open-ended questions.*

Beware too many choices—such as "What do you want for breakfast?"—as too many options and/or a lack of structure can feel overwhelming (see Chapter 7) and pave the way for a possible power struggle ("I want cake").

DO extend choices to less central parts of the activity.

It's possible (not to mention both fun and productive) to build in less obvious choices, for the sole purpose of allowing your toddler to feel more autonomous. At the same breakfast, you might inquire whether your toddler wants to have her eggs on a plate or in a bowl, use the purple or green fork, try to sit down all by herself or have you help her, or sing "Row, Row, Row" or the "Muffin Man" while the waffle is in the toaster. You're probably way ahead of me here: this is a right-before-a-tantrum variation on the creativity theme that I encouraged you to weave into your general approach to reducing tantrums with your toddler or preschooler. The more creative you can be, the more parts of the meal can be structured into choices for your child; if enough are provided, you will be able to keep her from feeling as though she has no say in breakfast, a feeling that often paves the way for a tantrum to occur.

During the Tantrum: You're in It, So Now What?

The prevention strategies described above are tremendously helpful, but not all tantrums can be prevented. So now you're in it. Your toddler has gone boneless and is sprawled crying across the floor. What now?

At this point in the tantrum timeline, my number-one recommended strategy is:

Be Present and Listen

In some ways, this sounds deceptively simple. If you walked into a room and saw a father using this strategy with his son, you'd see a child having a tantrum—yelling, crying, maybe kicking the floor—and a man just sitting there with him. How hard could that be? Very, it turns out.

👍 DO just sit there—empathically.

In Western culture, we very rarely sit still and just listen to anything, let alone a wailing child. Our instinctive parental urge is to make the tantrum stop. We bend over backwards going through the different strategies one by one, just waiting for something—anything—to "work." And if nothing "works" to calm our child down, we do the next best thing for our own comfort: we check out a bit. We walk away, take out our phone, or start to do something else. All we want in that moment is for the crying, the yelling, and the kicking to stop; if that doesn't happen, whatever we tried didn't "work."

The other definition of something that "works," though, is something that makes our child *feel* better, something that's comforting in the moment. Sometimes a parent's presence—his ability to sit and *be* with all of the distress *without* trying to cut it short—is what a child needs. As explained in Chapter 2, tantrums are often a discharge of sorts, a catharsis of overwhelming emotions, and often the most "effective" thing a parent can do may be to sit near her child and nonverbally communicate her unconditional presence.

"Wait a minute," you're thinking. "You're contradicting yourself. When you were talking about strategic attention, you said not to give children too much attention when they're throwing tantrums. Now you're saying to sit by their side and be with them as they completely melt down? That doesn't make sense!" And you're right. Well, about everything except the not making sense part. It *does* make sense. Because, for better and worse, handling tantrums is more art than science. Not all meltdowns are the same, nor are all children. It may be that most of the time your toddler's tantrums occur because she gets a lot of attention for them. In that case, using "strategic attention" will likely be effective—much of the time. Once in a while, though, the same toddler may be on the verge of a tantrum because her feelings are not being heard; when that happens, "validating feelings" will be the way to go. And when she just needs to let some emotion out? Well, that's when "be present and listen" is your best bet.

DO distinguish between feelings and behaviors.

As your child is letting out all of her feelings, it may be that she becomes so overwhelmed—by anger, frustration, distress—that she engages in certain behaviors that are not OK, namely those that are not safe for her or those around her. These might include hitting, kicking, scratching, or hurling wooden blocks across the room. At this point, you need to make a distinction between her feelings and her behavior, with the underlying message being that although all feelings are welcome in your home, all behaviors are not: "Chloe, I see that you are so angry. You can yell and scream and cry and kick the floor as hard as you can, but I will not let you hurt me [or your little sister, or the dog]. That is not OK."

DO use a firm—not angry—tone of voice.

Ideally, your presence—including your words and actions—will ultimately help soothe your child; we want him to experience you as both loving and containing. When you use words like the ones in the previous paragraph, speak firmly, in a way that conveys you are setting an important limit, but not one that communicates your own anger and frustration. Might you feel angry and frustrated? Of course. Might you even *say* that you feel angry and frustrated? That too is OK (although it might be communicated more effectively after the eye of the storm has passed). Speaking in clearly angry tones, however, (including yelling) will have the opposite effect from what you intend; your child's emotion—anger, frustration, perhaps even guilt at this point—will escalate, and therefore so will the tantrum.

DO consider using touch to keep your child and yourself safe.

Sometimes your voice will not be enough to calm your child down, and you will be sufficiently worried about your or his safety that you need to respond physically. If your child tends to feel calmer when you place a hand on his shoulder or move closer to him, or even envelop him in a bear hug, then these are all options you can employ, although heed his cues as to whether this is something he actually wants or needs (as you likely know from your own experiences of strong feelings, sometimes physical touch from a loved one is welcome; other times it feels intrusive). Of course, if safety is an issue, then this of course comes first, and holding your little one in such a way that he does not hurt himself or anyone else is a priority regardless of his reaction (if safety is an ongoing concern during your child's tantrums, then, as suggested in Chapter 1, professional assistance is recommended). When thinking about the use of physical touch, pay attention to whether your child seems to receive more hugs and loving touch from you during a tantrum than at other times of day, as, once again, you don't want to fall into the trap of inadvertently rewarding (and thereby encouraging) the tantrum behaviors. If this is the case, make a conscious effort to up your physical affection at times when your child is not in the throes of a meltdown.

DO make keeping yourself calm a priority.

Whatever you do to keep yourself emotionally regulated—deep breathing, feeling into your body, reminding yourself that your little one's brain isn't yet fully cooked—now is the time to go for it. If you can exude calm and stability, your child will be able to use this to bring herself back into a regulated state. For me, this is sometimes as simple as listening to Van Morrison's "Into the Mystic"; when this song is on—right from the opening guitar chords—it is physically impossible for me to feel agitated. Thanks to Spotify and Sonos, I can (and have been known to) play this song while one of my kids is mid-meltdown, in an effort to bring myself to a calmer place.

 Q "How do I know when it's OK to give in? You said it's OK once in a while, but I don't want to send the wrong message to my kid."

 A How I wish I could be precise or mathematical about this, providing some algorithm by which you'll always know when it's OK to give in and when it's not. So often, I have clients who ask me this very question, who fear inconsistency, and possibly reinforcing their children's tantrums, more than anything else. I'll tell you what I tell them. First: relax. Truly. Because there's actually no such thing as the "right" time to give in and the "wrong" time to give in. There's simply a choice point—one of thousands—and all you can do as a parent is take an action and then deal with the ramifications of that action. No one action—no matter how "wrong" or regrettable—is going to be the single determining factor in whether your child learns to behave in a certain desirable or undesirable way. There will be hills and valleys. You're shooting to trend positive, that's all. Second: the more you practice being present and attuned to your particular child, a theme that will come up again and again in this book, the easier this decision will be to make. Because, ideally, you want this to be a decision, a calm and intentional choice to act a certain way. If you are frequently giving in from a place of anxiety, or desperation, or resentment, then chances are there are some more effective strategies that would benefit both you and your child. This doesn't mean that once in a while you won't (gently) shove your child into his car seat with a "Fine, here's my phone!"—especially when you *really* need to get somewhere—but it does mean that this is not the kind of giving in we tend to strive for.

A quick personal anecdote here. A couple of nights ago, Henry called me into his room at 3:11 A.M. to ask for more ice in his water. 3:11 A.M. More. Ice. In. His. Water. He was thirsty, and doesn't like it when the water in the sippy cup by his bed isn't "super cold," it seems. I said no and intended to hold firm on this, given the absurdity, to my mind, of his request. But then he started pitching a fit. And he was half asleep. And he wasn't heeding my warnings that his yells could wake up his brother. And I was exhausted, and had a really busy schedule the following day. And so I caved. Except, in that moment, it didn't feel like caving, because it was a conscious choice to weigh the different factors and choose what felt like my best option in that moment. And so I said exactly that: "Henry, I just changed my mind. I am going to get more ice for your water, because it's really important to me that we both go back to sleep—that feels like the most important thing right now." And that's my final point on this question. I always recommend that if and when you give in to your child's demand, you explain that you changed your mind, so that your child knows that it was not his or her behavior that led to the outcome. Now, the jury's out as to when they actually understand that piece, but it feels good—and is good practice—to say it. It also provides some transparency as to the way you make decisions, which can be helpful to model for kids. The good news is that Henry hasn't called me in again to address predawn beverage temperature concerns, but I was aware that he might, and was prepared to handle the consequences. It was one choice point. I chose a path. That's all you can do.

After: Repair and Reflect

At this point in our timeline, your little one has stopped heaving, although maybe he's still breathing heavily. His tears have been wiped with a tissue or a sleeve (his or yours). What happens now?

 DO repair the rupture.

This is where it's helpful to invoke the concept of rupture and repair, first introduced in Chapter 6. For all intents and purposes, a tantrum is a rupture in the parent–child relationship, no matter how brief or minor. Which means that ideally it's followed with a repair, or reconnection. There's no prescription for what this looks like, and it certainly doesn't have to be a huge deal. A repair can range from a simple "connect and redirect" ("Wow, that was a tough couple of minutes; come here, let's go read a book together") to a hug, to making a joke you both laugh at. More than anything else, it's an opportunity for you to send the message that big feelings are OK and for you and your child to get back into sync. Sometimes it will happen quickly and naturally; other times—due to your emotional state and/or a logistical obstacle—you may have to take a break for a few minutes and consciously build in a repair a little bit later.

 DO apologize if you acted in a way you wish you hadn't during the tantrum.

See the strategy on apologizing earlier in this chapter. And keep in mind that I'm *not* suggesting you apologize for your child's meltdown: "I'm so sorry Mommy made you cry, honey." We are never responsible for other people's—even our own children's—emotions and reactions. But if you failed to label and reflect your child's feelings ("Oh, come on; it's not that big a deal! You're totally overreacting!") or you yelled at your child ("Just stop it already! Enough!"), then it can be really meaningful to apologize for that. (Note: we all do it—see the koala parable in Chapter 9.)

 DO use the tantrum as an opportunity for reflection.

Every tantrum is an opportunity for us, as parents, to learn and grow. Was this particular episode unavoidable? Or might there have been a way to prevent the meltdown? If so, at what point in the chain (think back to the "chain analysis" in Chapter 2)? The more you incorporate this reflection into the tantrum timeline, the more easily the tantrum prevention skills will start coming to you, because reflection in the wake of one tantrum leads to forethought in the lead-up to another. Your capacity to understand, and be aware of, how tantrum interactions unfold between you and your child is directly linked to your ability, over time, to prevent and deescalate the episodes quickly and effectively.

In Summary: How We Spent Our Summer Vacation (a.k.a. More on the Power of the Pause)

Every summer, we go to Maine for a week with my entire extended family—Henry and Zeke get to spend time with their grandparents, uncles, aunts, cousins, great-uncles, great-aunts, and everyone's dogs. I still remember the epic tantrum that Henry threw there one evening in August 2016. On this particular night, not only did he not want to eat his dinner, but he wanted M&M's instead. Within seconds, he was in the middle of the kitchen floor shrieking, tears streaming, legs kicking hard against the wood floor. At home, I likely would have attempted to prevent and then deescalate his meltdown using various strategies described in the previous sections, ranging from reflecting his feelings to distraction to ignoring. In that moment, however, I took a quick inventory of the scene at hand, scooped Henry up in my arms, and took him outside to snuggle on the lawn. Might an observer have said that I was rewarding his behavior, that he might learn that screaming and kicking lead to attention and affection from Mom? Sure. But the key words here are *quick inventory*; in that moment, Henry's tantrum felt way more related to his extended overstimulation, coupled with a few days of being completely removed from his typical structure and routine. The M&M issue felt secondary, merely an external target on which his system could focus its complete overwhelm. Was my assessment correct? I don't know. The snuggling worked to calm Henry down, he never got his M&M's, and that was his last tantrum for about 36 hours. There's no way to know if a different approach would have yielded a similar outcome.

My ability to pause before responding to Henry, to take that quick inventory as he lost his mind on the kitchen floor, probably represented the most essential few seconds in this entire episode, way more than whatever strategy I ended up going with. It's in that pause that your power as a parent rests. In a mere second or two, you can size up what's going on with your child, check in with how you yourself are feeling, quickly survey the systemic influences at play (in this case: vacation, constant presence of extended family), and make a conscious and intentional choice about how to respond. It's *that* choice, that *conscious parenting*, and not the strategy itself, that sets the tone for all that follows.

Unfortunately (although I can think of some pros here as well), there is no one formula that will work to prevent or deescalate every tantrum for every child, which is why it sometimes seems like there is so much competing and even contradictory advice out there. As you come to the end of this chapter, don't try to zero in on the *one key strategy* that's going to cure your toddler or preschooler of tantrums once and for all. This is an impossible goal. Instead, think about how you might be able to better tune in to what's going on for your child at a given time so that you become more skilled at pausing to observe the interactions leading up to and during his or her tantrums. Over time and with practice, mixing and matching all of the strategies available to you will become more and more seamless.

Of course, it's also helpful, as you do this, to cultivate an awareness of what not to do, of the various "anti-tools" or approaches that can make toddler and preschooler meltdowns worse. We turn to these "don'ts" in Chapter 9.

"Am I Making Things Worse?"

Concrete Ways to Avoid Knee-Jerk Responses and Other "Anti-Tools" That Just Don't Work

Dedicating a whole chapter to what *not* to do during a tantrum—the *don'ts*—sounds a bit like focusing on the negative, which is the opposite of what I typically advise (see "Using Attention Wisely" in Chapter 8; it's not just for kids!). But I've found it important to point out some specific tactics that, in my experience, many parents are inclined to use, to help you avoid them. They not only don't work but sometimes make things worse. Some of these may seem obvious, because they're the opposite of important *dos* discussed in Chapter 8 and also exemplified in other places in this book. Still, taking a moment to consider why it's particularly crucial to avoid them—with some tips on how to do so—can help cement your resolve not to turn to them reflexively.

👎 DON'T invalidate your toddler's perspective or emotions.

When parents describe their toddler's tantrums, they frequently speak in an incredulous tone. "You don't understand," they'll say. "She completely freaks out over the smallest thing!" Parents constantly use this word, "smallest," and the many synonymous words and phrases—"littlest," "most unimportant," "most trivial"—to describe the things that trigger their child's tantrums. There are whole memes and websites devoted to the idea, and for good reason; on their face, the reasons toddlers throw tantrums can be patently absurd. Last night I overheard Henry burst into tears while in the bath, and then heard my husband respond, "I'm sorry, Henry. I'm sorry that I took off your Band-Aid after you told me to take off your Band-Aid." Yes, you read that correctly. My husband was apologizing for doing exactly what it was that Henry had requested; for whatever reason, mere seconds later, Henry found it to be very upsetting. Or not what he expected. Or perhaps he had changed his mind. Or *something*. The fact is, I had no idea why Henry had burst into tears, and I laughed out loud (although not loud enough for Henry to overhear!) when I overheard my husband's sincere, if ridiculous on its surface, apology.

And yet, when we are with our little ones, it's important that we don't laugh, that we take their reactions and experiences seriously. Will you let out a giggle once in a while by accident? Of course. But looking at their distress from your own adult perspective only adds fuel to the fire. Some examples of invalidating reactions, aside from blatantly laughing at your child, include:

- "X is not a big deal." When in the history of the world has this ever worked with anyone? Your toddler or preschooler will never say, "You know what? You're right, Mom. It's totally not. My bad—blew it way out of proportion." Frankly, it's not just kids. No one responds this way. Ever.

- "Oh come on, it's only X." The "only" here is the big clue that you are patronizing your child by discounting whatever it is she's upset about. The word "just," in the same context, is also a giveaway. Be on the lookout for those words—*even when said in a seemingly empathic tone*—when your little one is falling apart.

- "There's nothing to get so upset about." Again, think about your own experiences with being upset. Is it ever helpful to be told you're upset for no reason? No. Either you believe there is a good reason to get so upset or you're aware of the absence of a "reason" from a logical standpoint, and yet you're upset anyway. And now you're also ashamed of being upset, since apparently there's nothing to get upset *about*. No matter how you cut it, this admonishment doesn't feel good and can even make things feel worse.

- "You're being ridiculous." This one pretty much speaks for itself. No one likes to be told he's being ridiculous, whether age two or 42. The same goes for words like "unreasonable" and "irrational." Plus, were some hyperverbal, super-insightful two-and-a-half-year-old ever to look back at his parents and respond, "Sure am! I'm a toddler!" he'd be right. After all, remember from Chapter 3 that your little one's brain is built in such a way that he's bound to be way more emotional than reasonable.

> Downplaying the importance of whatever is making your toddler melt down is favoring adult reason over toddler emotion, and it just won't work.

👎 DON'T tell your child how to feel.

This is a great general rule (to apply to toddlers, preschoolers, and the rest of humankind) and is particularly relevant for tantrums. It's certainly related to the idea of invalidation but goes one step further. These are comments that not only invalidate young children's emotions and experiences but also instruct them to feel something different than they do—for example, "Don't be angry," or "Stop getting so upset!"

I see this a lot around play, particularly when children are attempting to master a skill, such as constructing a building out of blocks or drawing a (more) perfect circle. Often, during these activities, children scream or cry when they "mess up," prompting parents to rush in to "help," also known as "do whatever it takes to avoid a meltdown." Parents immediately tell their child that there's "nothing to get upset about," or that they "can try again." I even had a parent tell her daughter how great it was that the dog had knocked down her perfectly assembled magnet-tile dollhouse because "now we get to have a super-duper fun time building it again!" Although these comments sometimes work to stave off a tantrum in the moment, I've often seen young children get even more upset in response. In contrast, however, they frequently calm down when parents simply help label their feeling or describe the circumstance at hand. "You're frustrated that it looks more like a rectangle than a circle, huh?" or "You were working so hard, and then the dog came over and ruined it." When children have the opportunity to have their emotions heard and understood by their parents, they feel soothed and no longer have to demonstrate their distress with louder screaming or harder crying. Once they're in the process of calming down, you can talk about how to proceed, whether that be rebuilding the dollhouse or taking a break from drawing circles.

If, on the other hand, they are told often enough not to feel what they feel, toddlers and preschoolers may come to believe that they have the ability to switch their emotions on and off on a dime or—more accurately—that they *should* be able to do so. And not only should they *have* this magical power, but they should exercise it not when *they* want to, but when their parents want them to. There can certainly be value in teaching (typically slightly older) children the power of positive thinking, or that our thoughts become our realities, or some other similar notion, but leading up to or during a tantrum is definitely not the time to do so. Young children need to learn that their feelings are part of life—even the difficult ones—and that they come and go, like waves in an ocean we need to ride (an analogy I didn't make up but often invoke). As parents, we need to model and teach them how to *cope* with these feelings (see Chapter 8), not how not to *have* them, which, frankly, won't work anyway. Also in this category: "Relax!" and "Calm down!" Just stop saying that. To everybody. Period.

🗲 DON'T avoid your child's difficult emotions.

This *don't* stems naturally from the first two, because—in my experience—it's the driving force behind them. If we didn't fear or, for some other reason, find it extraordinarily difficult to tolerate our children's distress, there would be many fewer instances of invalidating their emotions or demanding that they calm down or cheer up. Often, as described in Chapter 4, witnessing our children's distress brings up emotions or anxieties we experienced in our own childhoods; in the moment, it's not always easy to differentiate between what we felt then and what they feel now (which is when the mantras listed on page 77 can come in handy). And even if that's not the case, this reaction still makes perfect sense. I often think about the quote (attributed to different people) that having children is like having your heart walk around outside your body. It can feel like your heart will crack in two when you watch your child struggling in any way, including with feelings of anger, frustration, or disappointment. And yet there is no magic fairy dust that will prevent your child from ever feeling these things or, conversely, ensure that he is always happy. Parents frequently tell me that they have started to "walk on eggshells" for fear of setting off a tantrum. If you think about it, this will only serve to make tantrums worse when they do happen (which they will); not only will your little one be upset because she can't watch another episode of *Dora*, but she'll be upset because you have communicated that her tantrums are SO scary they are worth avoiding at all costs. No more *Dora* + terror that she is feeling the very feelings you have worked so hard to protect her from = more frequent and intense tantrums.

DON'T lie to your child to head off a tantrum.

This leads pretty naturally from the *don't* on the previous page, as often parents lie—or, ahem, tell half-truths—to avoid simply saying no and having their child experience (and express, likely in tantrum form) disappointment or frustration. Are there times when a little fib is OK? Yes. Once in a while, you can, of course, tell your toddler or preschooler that there are no more cookies, even though you know there's another unopened box in the pantry. But telling your child that the iPad is broken (when you just don't want him to use it) or that the toy store is closed (when you just don't want to stop there on the way home) doesn't do your child, or you, any favors. Well, that's not quite true. It does do you a favor in the short run, as the following 10 minutes will undoubtedly be easier than they might otherwise be. And occasionally you may—for whatever reason—need to prioritize those 10 minutes. But in the long run, getting in the habit of relying on these untruths sets a pretty lousy precedent. To put it bluntly, you're lying to your kid; there's really no way around it. You are supposed to be her most trusted person, and you're not being truthful. Remember the value of modeling? (If not, see Chapter 8.) If you want your child to be honest with you, you need to be honest with her. Because sooner or later she's going to realize that the iPad doesn't just spontaneously break at a certain time each day, and then what will she start thinking about all the other things you've been telling her? Children need to see parents taking responsibility for setting limits in an open and clear way, which means you need to practice.

 DON'T say that your child's behavior is making you sad.

I've heard this one a lot over the years. A child will begin to get angry or upset about something, and a parent will respond by making a sad face or pretending to cry, remarking, "You know it makes me so sad when you act like that." I've already said it, and I'm saying it again: *children are not responsible for their parents' emotional well-being.* This road goes in a single direction, and it's the other one: parents are responsible for their children's emotional well-being. Because of this, attempting to motivate your toddler's behavior by noting the effect on your feelings is a slippery slope. Will it be important for him to learn that his behavior affects other people? Of course. Nonetheless, it's developmentally inappropriate to ask that he act a certain way out of a sense of responsibility for your feelings. While we're on this topic, I'd cut the whole sentence construction—"you are making me feel X"—from

your interactions with your child more generally. The phrasing implies that your child
has a whole lot of power, which, as discussed
in Chapter 7, can feel overwhelming and
ultimately lead to anxiety. Saying "I am
starting to feel frustrated/angry/upset" is
preferable, as the wording implies that your
feeling states are your own and models your
ability to recognize and label them, then act
accordingly—a skill your child will benefit
from learning himself.

> Telling your child
> that his tantrum
> is making you feel
> sad might stop him
> in his tracks for a
> minute, but it won't
> last and puts a
> responsibility on his
> shoulders that he's
> not ready to carry.

*Modeling what you want to see from your
child is always happening and always important (see Chapter 8).*

👎 *DON'T take tantrums—and the things your little one says before
or during them—personally.*

Q-TIP is a great acronym (and one whose origin I don't know). That is: Quit
Taking It Personally. Write this down, laminate it, and hang it on the wall
in every room. Or set an alarm to go off on your phone that reminds you
of this every hour on the hour. When your toddler or preschooler is having
a tantrum, she may well pull out all the stops. What does that look like? "I
hate you!" "You're a bad mommy!" "I want Daddy, not you!" "Go away!"
"You're mean!" These things are never easy to hear, especially from your
own child. Depending on factors in your own past (as explored in Chapter 4), it may be very triggering for you to be the recipient of such direct
rage. And yet, as discussed in Chapter 3, these comments are appropriate
expressions of anger for children this age. Becoming angry and responding
in kind—"You're mean, too" or (I heard this once) "You're meaner"—does
nothing to help alleviate your little one's distress and will undoubtedly
escalate the situation. It also implies that the two of you—you and your
child—are expected to adhere to similar standards of behavior, which is
both false and confusing.

I also don't recommend commenting on your child's decorum or
manners in that moment—"Don't talk to me that way" or "Stop being so
disrespectful." Sure, your job is to teach your child to be respectful and
have good manners, but doing so in this way, at this moment, will almost
guarantee that he doesn't actually hear the message. After all, we—humans

of *all* ages—are notoriously bad at taking in new information when our emotions are running high. Responding in this way also opens the possibility for a power struggle about manners, which will only compound and intensify the tantrum already under way.

Of note, these comments—"I hate you," and so forth—can serve as a tantalizing invitation to invalidate your child's feelings, the number-one *don't* addressed on page 170. Parents often respond intuitively with what they know to be the case: "No you don't." Of course these parents are right in the larger scheme of things, because adults have the capacity to think in general terms and therefore look beyond the present moment. Remember, though, from Chapter 3, that young children can't yet do this, which is why one of the most important things parents can do to prevent tantrums is to see the world the way their child does (see Chapter 8). In that moment, your child *does* hate you—that is, she is the toddler version of very, very angry at you. As difficult as it may be, you're much more likely to head off or deescalate a tantrum by accepting and acknowledging that to be the case than by denying the overall veracity of the statement. (I offer some alternative responses in the Q&A at the end of Chapter 4.)

> Remember Q-TIP: Quit Taking It Personally.

 DON'T use sarcasm.

Although somewhat ubiquitous in this day and age, sarcasm is a rather sophisticated form of communication and one that young children are not able to understand. They may pick up on the fact that your tone doesn't match your words (such as when "very funny" is stated in a bitter or ominous way), but they won't know what to make of that. Sarcasm is frequently confusing for toddlers and preschoolers, as well as belittling. Some examples of sarcastic comments I have heard from parents leading up to or during their child's tantrum:

"Yes, and I want world peace."

"Your life is just *so* hard."

"I know! It's the end of the world!"

"Because [insert whatever here] is so clearly the most important thing on the planet."

Part of our job as parents is to model the kinds of communication we want our children to learn; think about this when you use sarcasm. Again, see the section on modeling in Chapter 8; few things are as important, not only when it comes to tantrum prevention but also with regard to parenting young children more generally. At best, your toddler or preschooler will feel confused by your use of sarcasm when he is upset. At worst, he will feel demeaned. Either way, it's an almost certain bet that his distress will go up and the tantrum will get worse and not better. (Similarly, little kids may "behave better" in the short run when they are a little afraid of their parents, but in the long run cultivating your child's fear of you to maintain some semblance of control is ineffective—and worse. See the Q&A on page 109.)

👎 DON'T threaten to call the police if your child becomes aggressive.

I think it goes without saying that you are not actually going to call the police if your three-foot-tall son hits his baby brother. If you are, we have bigger problems to address. Ideally (and of course I understand this is a complex sociopolitical issue and varies by community), our children grow up to trust, rather than fear, the police. Given that (1) you are not going to call the police, (2) the police would have a difficult time taking you seriously even if you did, and (3) as parents, it never serves us (let alone them) well to play on young little ones' fears, this is a tool to strike from your repertoire completely. Shots—as in, "If you keep acting this way, you are going to get a shot the next time you go to the doctor!"—also fall into this category, for reasons I hope are obvious by now.

👎 DON'T expect your children to be grateful for all they have.

Although this falls under the general heading of having realistic developmental expectations, it merits its own focus, given how frequently many of us have these thoughts. "How can my child get so upset about not getting another cookie? There are children starving in so many parts of the world!" or "I can't believe my child asked why there weren't any more birthday presents after opening all the ones she got; I was so embarrassed!" Issues around gratitude and privilege are complicated, in different ways, for parents from a range of backgrounds, which is why they are an explicit area of focus in Chapter 4. And yet this is a key area where we need to keep in mind where our little ones are developmentally, particularly when it comes to their egocentrism, as highlighted in Chapter 3. For the most part, your child doesn't (or is only just beginning to) understand that everyone's experience isn't like hers (or her friends'). Again, this is simply a function of this stage of brain development. Even when your child is old enough to understand this reality, though, hammering home the lesson that she needs to feel pure and constant gratitude for her abundance may lead to experiences of guilt or anxiety if (and, inevitably, when) she does not.

I once worked with a father who felt enormously proud of the fact that his four-year-old daughter was acutely aware of the many advantages she had been given in life. She spoke regularly about how lucky she was to go to private school, get three meals a day, and have two parents who loved her. All of these things did, in fact, make her quite lucky, and it was understandable that her father wanted to foster a sense of gratitude in her. The problem, however, is that if you attempt to instill this message too early, too forcefully, or—as pertains to tantrums—at a time when your child is upset about something comparatively trivial or superficial, you are essentially denying her the opportunity to ever be in a bad mood, to feel crappy about anything. Not surprisingly, this father's grateful little girl often seemed quite overwhelmed by her feelings of frustration or disappointment, possibly because she felt guilty for having them in the first place, given her knowledge of her overall good fortune. I can't say for certain, of course, but I do know that when her father stopped highlighting her good fortune so much, her emotional meltdowns became less frequent and intense. At the risk of being redundant, the most effective way to instill in our young children the values and skills that are important to us is to model these skills and values ourselves. For more on ways to model gratitude check out the "Parenting and Family" section of *Greater Good Magazine*, published by the Greater Good Science Center at the University of California–Berkeley (link listed in the Resources at the back of the book).

👎 DON'T call your child names.

OK, I know (or certainly really hope) you're not calling your toddler or preschooler an idiot or stupid or anything like that. But there are other, more subtle ways to call children names that can be damaging as well. Sometimes I hear parents call their little ones selfish or mean in the lead-up to or during a tantrum. These labels are harsh assessments of emotions and behaviors that often are not in our children's control. Remember our discussion in Chapter 3: toddlers and preschoolers are impulsive, rigid, egocentric, and emotional. They value control over most other things. In adults, some combination of these characteristics may well be considered mean or selfish; were you setting someone up on a blind date, this profile of her potential dinner companion would surely make her run for the hills. If we keep in mind child development, however, we come back to the idea that these behaviors are normal and expected of young children. When we call them mean or selfish, we're not only unfairly judging them according to adult standards but shaming them for being who they are and exactly who they're supposed to be. The result? Quite likely more tantrums.

In addition to mean and selfish, I've frequently heard parents refer to their children as:

- So emotional/intense
- A crybaby
- Dramatic
- An actor/actress
- Faking it

Now, there are times when young children do act out emotions purposely; they might pretend to cry or be upset as part of their ongoing attempt to understand how feelings and reactions work. Typically, these are nice, connected moments; you might tell your two-and-a-half-year-old that it's time for bed, and she'll "fake cry," then look at you and smile. Similarly, she might instruct you in pretend play: "You cry when I take away your toy, OK?" These are examples of little ones engaging in exploration—of feelings, roles, reactions—and they are not what I am referring to here. I'm also not referring to parents who describe their child as intense or very emotional in warm tones, with an understanding of his temperament and therefore his needs (see Chapter 5).

No, in these cases, I am talking about when a child is clearly experiencing genuine frustration, disappointment, anger, or sadness—*even if her reaction appears exaggerated in order to evoke a response*—and a parent responds by noting the child's "acting skills" or "flair for the dramatic." Has anyone ever told you—or even implied—that your distress about a particular situation wasn't real? That you were overreacting or faking it to get what you want? It feels really, really bad. It probably made you feel even worse than you were already feeling, and therefore you got even more upset. The same is true for our young children.

👎 *DON'T give negative consequences—including time-out—*
for tantrums.

Once again, here's the thing—and just because I've already said this over
and over doesn't mean I'm not going to keep saying it—tantrums are developmentally appropriate and normal expressions of strong emotion. Sometimes they are calls for communication and connectedness. Other times
they are attempts to test limits, to ensure that a solid structure exists and
will remain sturdy and in place. Still other times, they are reflections of a
trigger or unresolved issue on your part as a parent or a recent change in
your family system or larger environment. Tantrums can be a lot of things.
What tantrums cannot be are punishable offenses that will decrease if followed
by a negative consequence, such as a time-out or removal of privileges. Tantrums
themselves are made up of several discrete and overlapping behaviors;
although you may work on discouraging some (such as through the use
of strategic attention, as discussed in Chapter 8), you will never be able to
keep tantrums as a whole from occurring. To that end, putting in place a
negative consequence (time-out or removal of privileges) specifically for a
tantrum is not going to be effective and may even be shaming. This is not
to say that removing your attention (ideally following a kind, empathic
remark) cannot be a useful strategy (as discussed in Chapter 8), as your
child may need a break to calm down and pull himself together. Having
this be the purpose of the break—allowing him to learn to cope with, and
regulate, his emotions versus some kind of punishment—is essential. (For
more on tantrums and time-outs specifically, see the Q&A on page 106.)

I want to draw your attention to the fact that "lose your temper" did
not make this list of *don'ts*. Does this mean that I recommend your completely losing your temper the next time your toddler has a meltdown? Of
course not (it didn't make the *do* list either, after all). But the reason I didn't
include it here is that at some point—maybe not tomorrow or next week—
you will. And what's more? At some point you already have. You raised your
voice louder than you meant to, or said something you still regret. Even
after you finish this book, you'll find yourself back there again; you'll take
a nasty tone with your little one, or somehow let a curse word slip out. A
friend once called me early in the morning: "Please tell me I didn't damage
Thea forever," he begged, only half joking. His three-year-old had asked
for her adored stuffed koala bear 90 minutes into a pre-bedtime tantrum.
"Here's your f*&$ing koala!" he had said, and thrown it at her. I reassured

him that his daughter would be OK; this was a few years ago, and I'm happy to report she is indeed thriving.

I wasn't surprised, of course, that this dad—typically quite skilled and tuned in as a parent—had lost it during bedtime, as that's when so many of us do. Bedtime is among the trickiest times of day when it comes to preventing tantrums, although it has several notorious partners in crime, including mealtimes and bath time, among others. Chapter 10 provides specific strategies aimed at increasing your (and your child's) chances of survival when it comes to heading off tantrums during these well-known witching hours.

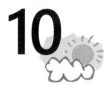

10

"Please Just Go to Sleep, Already!"

How to Reduce Tantrums at Tough Times of Day, from Wake-Up to Bedtime

Every parent knows that not all parts of the day are created equal when it comes to tantrums. Certain hours of the day run like clockwork, so much so that you momentarily forget how practiced your toddler or preschooler has become at her Jekyll and Hyde routine. Other hours feel like days, dragging on painfully with meltdown after meltdown, as you watch your last ounce of sanity disappear in a mess of tears, snot, and drool (your little one's certainly, but sometimes yours too). Although which hours fall into which category depends a little bit on the particular child and parent, most families with young children have some difficult times of day in common. I've compiled them in the following pages, along with my best shot at "quick tips" to pull you through. (Please do use these as short-term work-arounds—we all need them sometimes—but don't forget that the work of calming tantrums is most effective when it blends immediate pragmatic tools like these with concepts like love and limits and a deeper dive into child development and self-reflection, all of which are presented earlier in the book. If you run into the mention of a strategy that you'd like to know more about, you might not have read Chapter 8 yet and can refer to the more detailed descriptions of strategies there.)

Early in the Morning

Here's a somewhat obvious point that often gets overlooked: many young children are not morning people. Sure, some get up raring to go, roadrunner-style. But others need time and space to wake up, adjust to daylight, and come to terms with another rotation of the planet on its axis. A lot of tantrums happen first thing in the morning because of the mismatch here. Parents need to start their morning routine, and so they pummel their child with questions and commands before she is fully ready. Within seconds of her getting out of bed, Mom is throwing out a string of information her little brain can't yet process: "Come here! Give me a hug! How'd you sleep? What do you want for breakfast? Today you have music class! Let's go pee-pee!" A toddler who's just waking up may feel overwhelmed by all the input, and feeling overwhelmed can easily result in a tantrum. Alternatively, there may be a preschooler who wakes up and is off to the races, but it's the parent who's precoffee, and thus preverbal. This child has a list of demands before the sun is even up; when Dad can barely understand let alone meet them, this too can result in a tantrum of the before-breakfast variety.

Once everyone is up and about, the real fun starts; mornings are a high-demand time: there are a lot of things your child has to do that he probably doesn't want to (brushing teeth is a biggie). There are also a lot of things you have to do that you probably don't want to (such as get ready for work or do anything other than sleep seven more hours). Your child's needing to do things he doesn't want to + your needing to do things you don't want to + a ticking clock + lingering exhaustion (certainly on someone's, but possibly on everyone's, part) = fertile ground for tantrums. Given that we can anticipate this, how do we empower ourselves to bypass the early-morning tantrum train (remember, anticipation = empowerment)?

> Most families' early-morning schedule is a formula for disaster in the form of tantrums.

1. *Do what you can to make sure your child has slept long and well the night before.* Easier said than done, I know. Also not a primary focus of this book. Sleep continues to deserve mention, however, due to its extreme importance and link to tantrums. Again, please see the Resources in the back of the book if you need help in this area.

2. *Think structure and routine*—also beginning the night before. If there are morning tasks that can get done the night before (making the child's lunch if she needs to take it to preschool, picking out clothes, for her and/ or for you, etc.), do them. The more relaxed you are in the morning, the more present you can be to tune in to your child and meet him where he is

with regard to mood and energy level. Note the interplay here between love and limits; focusing on the latter in advance ensures you can maximize the former when it's needed most.

3. The point in the previous paragraph needs highlighting, so much so that I'm giving it its very own place on this list: *meet your child where he or she is with regard to mood and energy level.* Tricky times of day are when you need to "get" your child, as described in Chapter 6, most of all. The interactions you have with your child first thing in the morning will set the tone for the next hour, if not the entire day. If your child seems grumpy and out of it, don't come at him in full-on camp counselor mode, of either the nonstop fun or the taskmaster type. Rather, let him warm up a bit, speak in quiet tones, feel him out, follow his lead. If your child seems ready to take on the world, do your best to muster some enthusiasm for his plans, answer his questions, and join in his enthusiasm about the day ahead instead of "yucking his yum" (being a downer).

If the latter seems impossible—your child wakes up with the energy of a new puppy every morning, and you barely remember your own name until you've had caffeine—then choose another, nonmorning time to talk about this and come up with a plan that works for both of you. One client of mine, Hannah, explained to her constantly-full-of-beans three-year-old, Jason, that she always needed five minutes after she woke up just to herself, that the "Mommy alone time" was really important so that she could then have fun "Mommy–Jason time." Jason had an ingenious idea (as three-year-olds often do); what if, during those five minutes, he completely disappeared? And so, the perfect morning game for their family was invented. When Hannah got out of bed, she set a timer, at which point Jason would hide. When the timer went off five minutes later, Hannah would look for Jason; when she found him, they'd share a morning hug and get on with the day. The daily tantrums that had been occurring—when Jason infringed on Hannah's space, leading Hannah to feel claustrophobic and frustrated, leading Jason to feel blamed and rejected—basically ceased, having been replaced by a calm, connected start to the day that worked for everyone.

4. Have a *morning routine* in place for all of the tasks that need to be accomplished—not just in your head, but written out and hung on the wall (with pictures, so your little one can "read" it). List all the things your child needs to do in the morning (get out of bed, use the potty/toilet, have breakfast, brush teeth, get dressed, brush hair, put on socks/shoes, etc.). Point to the corresponding picture as you do each one, and, if she is old enough,

maybe use a whiteboard so she can check the tasks off as she goes. (Pinterest and Etsy are great for ideas on how to get creative with making visuals for kids' schedules/routines.) Here are some ideas that take advantage of the *do*s in Chapter 8:

- For each task at hand, use strategic attention, commenting on what your child *is* doing rather than *is not* doing.
- Build in choices, so that your child feels the autonomy he craves. Does he want to use the purple or the green bowl for his cereal? Does he want to wear the red socks or the blue socks?
- Introduce songs, games, contests, or races to make things fun instead of boring or effortful. Putting on pants doesn't exactly scream excitement. Seeing who can put pants on first, you or Mommy, is a huge improvement.
- Include favorite toys/objects to help your cause. (Your teddy bear would love to watch you brush your teeth, no doubt! Shall we bring him? After we brush yours, we can brush his!)
- Be ready with distraction/humor. For example, turn the situation on its head with an unexpected twist by asking your toddler or preschooler to help *you* put your shoes on or brush your teeth.
- Introduce a daily reward that can be put into place when and only when all of the tasks have been completed. Ideally, this is a reward that makes sense from a time perspective and that reinforces your child's desire to move through the morning tasks efficiently. So, for example, if your child completes what she needs to do, she will have time to play, or time to have a bit of screen time, or time to do a special errand with Daddy on the way to preschool.

> A picture schedule can make your family's morning routine stay, well, routine (no tantrums).

Leaving the House

If your home houses one or more young children, then leaving can feel like biking in the Tour de France, or climbing Mount Everest, or doing whatever monumental-thing analogy you prefer. It's also a notorious time for tantrums. Why? First, our own expectations, introduced in Chapter 4, play a large role here. Most notably, parents tend to expect leaving the house to be a shorter activity than it actually is. For adults, the act is simply a means to an end. When toddlers and preschoolers are involved, however, leaving the house is an activity unto itself. I see this in my practice all the time. A parent will need to drop her little one at day care by, say, 8:45 A.M. to make it to work on time. It takes 15 minutes to get to day care from home, so said parent will plan to leave the house at 8:30 A.M. "What time," I will innocently ask, "does that mean you have to start leaving the house?" Often I am met with a puzzled expression. "What do you mean, *start* leaving?"

I have never met a family with a young child who can get from "Come on, honey; it's time to go" to "Excellent, now we're out the door!" in under 10 minutes (at the absolute minimum). Leaving the house is a process, one that's made up of more individual components than you may realize: shoes have to go on (you, your little one, spouses and siblings if present/involved), you have to find your fill-in-the-blank (purse, wallet, keys, phone, train ticket, Metrocard), you have to make sure you have your fill-in-the-blank for your little one (lunch, snack, diapers, wipes, cream, tissues, toy, book, weird-object-of-current-affection), you may or may not have to put him in a jacket (depending on season, geographical location—yes, this is a big reason to live somewhere tropical), you may or may not have to put him in a stroller or car seat, you may or may not have to turn out the lights, you may or may not have to lock the door, and so forth. Families differ on the specifics, but it's always a lot, and we never allot (pun intended) quite enough time, given the multiple tasks at hand. *When there's A LOT to do, ALLOT more time* (that one I can take credit for).

> Think of leaving home not just as a transition but as an activity or process if you want to discourage potential tantrums.

Second, leaving the house is a transition, and transitions are notoriously difficult for toddlers and preschoolers. It can be very difficult for them to "shift set," which is to say, go from one activity (for example, playing or eating breakfast) to another (leaving the house). This is a skill that comes with executive functioning, which is housed in the prefrontal cortex of the brain, an area only just beginning to develop in young children (see Chapter 3). Finally, leaving the house typically (albeit not always) occurs because there is some kind of obligation/time commitment about which parents are anxious, if not at first, then certainly increasingly as time ticks away. Parents need to get to work by a certain time, or a child needs to get to preschool or a class, or someone has a doctor's appointment, or there is a list of errands that need to get done before a particular time—the possibilities are endless. Young children, of course, have no sense of time's existence or importance, and so don't understand the need to rush. Parents become more and more tense, impatient, and brusque the closer it gets to the time when they "absolutely have to leave right this minute!"

 "My little girl always moves so incredibly slowly. Honestly, the bulk of her tantrums seem to be because we need to rush her to get places, and she just won't move any faster than she wants to!"

 Yes, toddlers and preschoolers move slowly. They are constantly looking around, or exploring, or playing some kind of game in their head that prevents them from getting a move on when you need them to ("Mommy, I need to wait at the top of the steps for the *dragon* to tell me I can move—not you, the *dragon*."). Furthermore, as discussed in this chapter, they don't have a real concept of time (no matter how much we want them to!), and once they know it's important to us to get somewhere, they may deliberately move even slower so as to exert their own control over the situation. This chapter discusses the importance of building in enough time for transitions, as well as some more specific strategies for handling this behavior, including games, races, and so on. What I want to say here, though, is more global, and perhaps even a bit revolutionary: I think our little ones have a lot to teach us grown-ups about how to move slower. Are there times we absolutely have to get somewhere? Of course. But there are also plenty of times when we don't, but act like we do nonetheless. Will it matter if we arrive 15 minutes later to a playdate? Or if we get to the playground a full hour after we planned because we enjoyed the walk there instead? It won't, and in these situations it's us, and not our children, who are guilty of being unnecessarily rigid. Sometimes toddlers and preschoolers are right to look at the world with curiosity and awe; it's we who have, sadly, forgotten to do so. The other day I was shuffling my kids in from the car to have dinner, when Henry pointed out the sunset. "Look how beautiful it is, Mommy." He was right. And I thanked him for slowing me down enough to notice.

Put all of this together, and it's a recipe for tantrums. Once again, because there's so much that has to get done, many demands are made of your toddler or preschooler—do this, don't do that, wait here, come with me, hurry up. High-demand situations even by themselves tend to lead to high-defiance situations, which, in turn, lead to power struggles that result in tantrums. Add to this, though, young children's difficulty transitioning, parents' high tension level, and not enough time allotted in the first place, and it's a near certain bet that a meltdown is coming down the pike. Helpful strategies:

1. Again, because it bears repeating (and perhaps even a sign on your fridge or Post-It on your mirror), *anticipation = empowerment*. When it comes to leaving the house, this can mean a few things. Most important, allot more time. *A lot to do = allot more time.* Build in at least a 15-minute cushion for leaving the house when planning your day.

2. Have a visual by the door with pictures of the different things that have to get done in order to leave.

3. Practice! Seriously, pick a mellow, nonrushed time to practice leaving the house with your child. Make it a fun activity, a game. The more young kids practice something, the better they get (which, of course, goes for older children and adults too).

4. Give your little one several warnings—say ten, five, and two minutes—before you need to start the leaving the house activity. Do this verbally, hold up your fingers, set a timer, or do all three. Make sure your child hears and understands the warnings (read: do not simply yell out, "five minutes!" from down the hall and expect this information to get absorbed and translated in all the right ways).

5. Have a song you always sing when it's time to leave the house, much like the famous "Clean-up" song that signals cleaning up to every toddler and preschooler in the nation. The song may be about leaving the house (should you know, or write, one of those), but doesn't have to be. Regardless, your child will come to associate the particular song with the activity at hand (in this case, leaving the house!).

6. Label and reflect feelings by:
- Saying something like "It seems like you're feeling a little frustrated, huh? Like you really don't want to stop what you're doing. It stinks to have to leave when you're having so much fun."

- Drawing on favorite toys/objects to describe the situation: "Your fire truck knows you have to go; he's sad, but can't wait to play with you later."

- Talking to the activity as if it were a character: "I hate you, Teddy Transition!" Or, "Why are you always making me stop playing, Have-to-Leave Lauren!"

7. Make sure to be aware of the strategic attention principle here. If your little one learns that her tantrums—or behaviors that lead to tantrums—postpone leaving the house when she doesn't want to, she will learn to continue those behaviors. This is often at play when it comes to putting on shoes or jackets: Does your toddler get more of you when she does or does not put them on when you ask?

8. Take a look at what leaving the house—especially at a certain time of day, say, morning—means for your toddler or preschooler. For example, does it always mean he's going to day care and you're off to work? If so, you'll want and need to address the role that impending and inevitable separation may be having in the tantrum interactions. Think back to Mia in Chapter 6, whose meltdowns at preschool dropoff got increasingly worse as her relationship with her mother, Pam, became more and more ruptured. When tantrums seem potentially related to separation, zeroing in on the "love" factor and increasing connectedness in and surrounding those moments is frequently a good place to start.

Mealtimes

Not surprisingly, meals and tantrums often go hand in hand for young children, for many of the same reasons we've discussed. First, toddlers and preschoolers are typically hungry around mealtimes, and crankiness can go up when blood sugar is down. Second, parents are often extraordinarily invested in their toddlers' eating for all kinds of reasons, including—at the core—that our number-one job is to keep our kids healthy, and nutrition is a huge part of that. Many parents work hard to prepare food for their kids and have expectations for how the food will be received; when little ones subsequently reject the food, parents take it personally, which raises the stakes and, thus, the likelihood of a tantrum interaction. Remember the wise words from Chapter 4: "Expectations are resentments under construction." Third, mealtimes with young children can be fraught because food is often a fraught topic for grown-ups (eating, body image, etc.); as always in these cases, kids pick up on this general energy. Fourth, like the other times of day described in this chapter, mealtimes are high-demand situations (where toddlers are given a lot of direction in a short period of time) and often necessitate a transition away from another, preferred activity. Finally, from a literal/physiological standpoint, it is impossible to force another human being to eat, and young children know this. They know that, no matter how much you want them to eat, they are in charge of their intake, and once grasped, this is an incredibly exciting realization that they will milk to no end. After all, as discussed earlier, there are few things toddlers and preschoolers crave more than control; only rarely does food make the cut.

For all of these reasons (and no doubt some I've neglected), mealtimes can be really tough with young children, and, not surprisingly, a lot has been written elsewhere on this topic (see the Resources for further guidance). A quick caveat before I get to some concrete pointers, which is that they apply primarily to toddlers and preschoolers who are, from a medical/physiological perspective, healthy, and whose pediatricians have voiced no concerns about their falling off their growth curve. For children with allergies or other conditions that may complicate eating and food intake, more individual guidance (with regard to nutrition and/or behavioral issues) is recommended. That caveat aside, here's what I can offer with regard to the infamous mealtime tantrums:

1. I subscribe to—and recommend to my clients—the "division of responsibility" put forth by the Ellyn Satter Institute, whereby the parent is in charge of the *what*, *when*, and *where* when it comes to food, and the child is responsible for *whether* and *how much*. That is to say, parents decide when mealtimes are, where they occur, and what is being served (for example, dinner is generally between 5:30 and 5:45 P.M. at the kitchen table, and on this particular evening you are serving chicken, pasta, and peas). Children then get to decide whether and how much they are going to eat of each item offered. This method has not only been shown to help children develop a healthy relationship with food (as in learning to read their body's cues/needs with regard to intake), but also, in my experience, vastly decreases the power struggles—and, thus, tantrums—that happen at the table. If you too opt to adopt this approach, make sure you always include at least one food that you know your child enjoys, so that you can ensure he doesn't walk away from the table hungry because he genuinely did not like any of what was available. Yes, this may mean that he eats only buttered pasta sometimes. This is a trade that I, and the majority of my clients, have been willing to make. The choice is, of course, yours and yours alone.

2. I confess: In our home, Henry frequently enjoys dessert as a palate cleanser, so to speak (where you might see grapefruit sorbet, he sees a Reese's Peanut Butter Cup). Yes, what I mean by this is that I often let him have his dessert halfway through dinner. Otherwise, as I learned the hard way, he asks for it nonstop and declares he is finished after only a few bites of his meal, when I know he is likely still hungry. Rather than engage in a power struggle in which he can only "earn" his sweets after he has taken a certain number of bites of his vegetables—potentially leading him to dislike foods he might otherwise enjoy—I let him eat his (predetermined and small) dessert whenever he wants. After he does, because there's no more anticipation (yes, this kid has a major sweet tooth) he typically eats a lot more of his actual food. We make sure to talk about how some foods are healthier than others, which is what influences how *much* we can have of each, but, to me, the order in which we eat them is not (as my husband is fond of saying) the hill I want to die on.

3. Check your own anxiety around eating issues. This is a huge area in which parents frequently need to do their own work to separate what's theirs from what's their child's, as discussed more generally in Chapter 4. I have worked with many families in which one or both parents needed to do some work on their own "stuff" around food, body image, or related issues before they were able to even begin to address their little one's tantrums at this time of day.

4. Along similar lines, when it comes to helping our children learn particular behaviors at mealtime, think modeling. If you yourself don't tend to try new foods, or sit for more than five minutes at a meal, it's a pretty sure bet that your toddler or preschooler will follow in your footsteps.

> Conflict at mealtimes can be reduced if you remember that these times are not strictly about nutrition.

5. Don't let food be the focus of mealtime! This may sound counterintuitive, but it shouldn't. Sure, we eat during meals, but that doesn't mean that the activity has to center around food. In part, if you follow some of the pointers already listed, this will be a natural by-product. A meal that consists only of talking and negotiating about food will be boring at best and miserable—for everyone—at worst. Ideally, mealtime is a fun, connected, time of family togetherness; research, in fact, suggests that eating together as a family is linked to various positive outcomes in children.

Although likely not possible (or desirable!) for every meal at this point, it's never too early to start laying the groundwork.

6. While not specifically about mealtimes, I want to include one quick note about snacks, which of course also fall under the eating/food heading. There are various approaches to snacks—if young children should be able to have them, if so at what time(s), what foods they should be allowed to have, and so forth. I am not going to go too far down that road because I don't want to stray too far from the topic at hand—tantrums. I will, however, simply say that one of my most popular recommendations is that parents decide on two to three snacks that their child is allowed to have at any time of day (perhaps with a few exceptions, such as within an hour of a meal or after teeth brushing at night). These include healthy foods that, frankly, from a nutritional standpoint, you don't really care if your child gorges on, typically fruits and vegetables (grapes, cucumber sticks, and frozen peas—wait, are my kids the only ones who like to munch on those?). You can even, if your child is closer to four or five years old, have a special place in the refrigerator where these are kept and which she is allowed to access at any time, thus granting her the autonomy she craves.

This way, as parents, you never need to worry that your child might actually be hungry if (or when) she is throwing a tantrum about wanting something to eat, which I have seen be a source of confusion for many parents over the years. If your child is genuinely hungry, she will be happy to have some fruit or veggies.

Bath Time

We can't have a chapter about tricky times of day without mentioning the bath. Some kids love getting in and hate getting out, other kids hate getting in and love getting out, still others hate getting in *and* getting out, and there are a whole bunch whose preferences change day to day, just to keep parents on their toes. Some of this is about water, although there is by no means a one-to-one correlation between those kids who love the bath and those kids who love swimming or water play. If your child's tantrums seem to be about a dislike of water, think about decreasing the frequency of baths. Unless your child has been dripping with sweat or running around in mud, or has finger-painted his stomach or actively stinks, a bath is not a necessity. In many countries, daily baths are unheard of. If a bath calms your child down before bed and is, therefore, a critical part of her wind-down routine, go for it. If, however, it's a source of frustration for everyone day in and day out, there's absolutely no medical or hygiene-related need to put your child (and yourselves) through that kind of torture. I have clients who claim my most life-changing suggestion was giving them permission to bathe their child only three to four times per week.

> Believe it or not, your child doesn't necessarily have to have a bath every single day.

Water aversion aside, by definition, both getting into and out of the bath represent transitions, and so everything said about transitions in this chapter applies here as well. And so many of the same strategies are recommended—games, contests, and races; reflecting feelings in various ways; telling "Becky Bath" that you're mad at her or are sorry you have to leave her behind until next time. In addition, consider:

1. Letting your child have control over the bath where possible, including:
   - Helping to set the temperature
   - Picking out the bathmat, washcloth, and towel
   - Having a voice in color/scent of shampoo/soap
   - Washing parts of her body by herself
   - Choosing order of what gets washed first, next, and so forth

2. Using toys/gimmicks to make bath time fun
   - Color tablets that change the color of the water
   - Bathtub paints and crayons
   - Bath toys his or her favorite theme/character
   - Bubble bath with favorite scents
   - Bath bombs

3. Preemptively using a timer to set the duration of the bath

4. Decreasing transitions where possible

For example, go straight from dinner to the bathroom and take off your little one's clothes there, rather than making a stop in her bedroom in between. Sounds like a small adjustment to make, and yet it removes a whole other setting (the bedroom) and two transitions (from dinner to

> For toddlers and preschoolers, fewer transitions = fewer opportunities for tantrums.

the bedroom and the bedroom to the bathroom) from the equation. As a general rule, decreasing the number of settings and transitions your child needs to navigate typically results in fewer opportunities for tantrums.

5. Showering together instead. Anyone up for a parent–child shower dance party?

Bedtime

We made it to bedtime! That is, the bedtime section of this chapter, which is distinct from bedtime in real life. That elation, though—that you've finally made it to the end of the day, that your child's sleep is right around the corner—is really important to note. Because, again, *our children can sense our energy*, and I've seen this dynamic completely transform what is ideally a calm, connected time to give closure to the day into a tantrum-filled nightmare. And when I say I've seen it, I mean over and over again with my clients, as well as—I'm not proud to say—in my own home with my own sons. That feeling of triumph when bedtime is nigh is undoubtedly familiar to all parents, whether it's an emotion you experience daily or just once in a while. Raising a child is hard work, and no matter how much we adore the little buggers, we can't deny that, at least some of the time, bedtime can't come soon enough. I've learned to accept rather than feel guilty about this (most of the time).

In my experience, the number-one—although not sole—reason that bedtime so frequently goes off the rails is that there's a disconnect between a tired child who craves connectedness and a parent who's too wiped out and impatient to provide it. At the very end of the day, before the separation that is nighttime, toddlers and preschoolers want to connect more than anything, and parents have pretty much had it; we're down for the count, checked out, thinking about what's next, how we will spend our imminent few minutes of precious alone time. In this way, we end up failing on the "love" side of things—not able to tune in and really *be* with our child—right at the time they need us most, while simultaneously often being too tired to provide clarity around the limits (the "OK, OK, fine, just one more book" syndrome). And so our little ones feel not seen and frustrated, unmoored and consequently not ready to bid the day farewell, and become all about pushing boundaries. Which we let them, because we're too tired not to, until we explode, and they explode, and boom: tantrum. What to do about this unfortunate cycle?

1. Do your best to get into a different mindset before bedtime. If it's going to go more smoothly and be free of tantrums, bedtime can't just be—in the words of so many of my clients—"something to get over with." Think of it as the final mile of a marathon, or a summit dash on a long mountain climb—that very last stretch of a strenuous journey during which, instead of backing off, you give it your all, dig down into your reserves, and expend energy you didn't even know you had. Only you know what you need to get into this headspace. Maybe it's picturing a running race or a rocky mountain, per the images suggested here. Maybe it's grounding yourself by taking a moment to feel your feet pressing into the floor. Maybe it's a deep breath, a mantra, a second with your eyes closed, a short body-scan meditation, or squeezing a pillow. *Right before bedtime, steal just a moment or two to do whatever will help you feel centered and regulated so that you can be present for and connected to your child.* Remember, he is little, and his brain has been working overtime. He needs help settling, and he looks to his connection to you for help with that. If you can't connect, or if you're unsettled yourself, he's for sure not going to be able to get to the calm and rested place he'll need to find so he can drift off to sleep.

> Toddlers and preschoolers need their connection with us to help them manage emotions and transitions, such as settling down so they can go to sleep.

2. You've heard it a million times before, and I'm going to say it again: *structure and routine* are critical here. Have a predictable set of activities you do each and every night before bedtime. Maybe you read a book or two or make up a story that stars your child as a character. Maybe you sing a favorite lullaby. Maybe you say good night to all of her family members and friends, one at a time ("Good night, Grandma; good night, Grandpa . . ."). Maybe you each say your favorite parts of the day. Maybe—especially if you've been away from each other all day—you list three different times you thought about her while you were gone, and what—*specifically*—you thought about (for example, "When I was eating my lunch, I thought about how you were probably eating your lunch at the exact same time and how I wished I

could wipe the crumbs off your chin and hear your giggle"). The point is to lay the groundwork for sleep not only by being calm and quiet, but also by restoring and highlighting the strong connection the two of you have.

3. Using *empathy* can be key at bedtime. Do you remember being little and your parents telling you to go to bed? It was the worst, right? At least some of the time? As parents of young children, it's nearly impossible to remember that going to bed was ever anything other than the epitome of pure bliss, but I promise this was once the case. When you're a child, there's so much exciting stuff in the world, so much to see and do and learn—it can feel like going to sleep is a waste of time, or that you'll miss out on more fun adventures, or that it would be so much more fun to be big and stay up late. If this is the sense you are getting from your little one, let him know you get it. Tell him a story about how you used to hate bedtime as a kid or give him a hug and say (something like) "It can be so tough to say good-bye to the day and to have to wait until tomorrow to play more. You want to stay up late and have more adventures! We'll have more adventures tomorrow, sweetie. Now it's time for sleeping."

4. Be prepared and structured about what needs to happen before you turn out the light (and sleeping in a dark room is highly recommended by sleep experts across the board). If your child is going to ask for water, have water there already. If your (potty-trained) child is going to say he needs to pee, using the potty/toilet should be part of the usual pre-bedtime routine, not an afterthought. If your child needs to sleep with fill-in-the-blank-here (which, for my kids, has ranged from pacifiers to stuffed animals, to six cars, to a straw hat, to a plastic bag of *Paw Patrol* characters, to a high-bouncer ball we got in the machine outside the diner), then make sure said thing is located and set up prior to lights out.

If you are having trouble setting limits around bedtime, remember that 10–12 hours of uninterrupted quality sleep is essential for toddlers' and preschoolers' health and brain development. The same way you wouldn't budge if he wanted gummy bears and chocolate for dinner, don't budge on this.

5. Don't fall into the common pitfall of letting your own fear of "creating a bad habit" stop you from connecting to your child authentically. In other words, if it would help bedtime to go more smoothly and be tantrum-free to sit on your child's bed (or reach down into her crib) and rub her back for a few minutes as she falls asleep, then it's OK to do that. I've seen several parents who have been so blindingly consumed

by what-if-she'll-never-be-able-to-fall-asleep-without-me panic that they've gone to completely unnecessary extremes on this, often missing out on an opportunity to soothe their child in a genuine way, thus paving the way for restful sleep (for everyone!).

And with that . . . you did it! You got through the day. You worked hard. Now go take a load off before another one starts in the morning. Because if there's one thing I can promise you, it's that morning will be here sooner than you think.

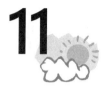

11

"How Many Times Can We Order Pizza for Dinner?" (a.k.a. Another Aborted Trip to the Supermarket)

How to Reduce Tantrums in Tricky Settings, from the Big-Box Store to the Playground and Beyond

Just as all times of day are not created equal when it comes to preventing tantrums, neither are all settings. A tantrum that begins the same way—say, with a few vehement *no*s and some stomping—may end very differently depending on whether your toddler is in your living room, your in-laws' living room, the playground, a supermarket, or a restaurant. Why? What are the ways in which a particular setting influences the trajectory of a tantrum? And, more important, what can we do about it?

As has been posited throughout this book, tantrums are, to a large extent, the product of interactions between young children and their parents or caregivers. And so when we are looking at the impact of place, or setting, on the nature and outcome of this dance, as it's described in Chapter 5, we need to look from the perspective of both participants—the child and the parent. Let's start with children.

How Some Places Set Toddlers and Preschoolers Up to Melt Down

For young children, new and unfamiliar settings can be overstimulating and potentially jarring or anxiety provoking in some way. And when toddlers and preschoolers feel like they can't get their bearings, and/or feel anxious or overstimulated, they can become overwhelmed and have more difficulty regulating their emotions.

Overwhelmingly New and Different

This can happen in all kinds of places, from the playground to "Mommy and Me" classes, from birthday parties to family gatherings or big-box stores (think Walmart, Costco, Target). The last is a great example: these stores are often overwhelming for grown-ups, so imagine how huge and maze-like and confusing they look to kids. Then put said kid in the front of a shopping cart with squeaky wheels that nearly topples when you navigate corners, and the result makes a tantrum a nearly sure thing. Of course, there are individual differences with regard to how different settings influence the likelihood, or intensity, of tantrums. For example, we can look at the role of temperament (discussed in Chapter 5). Some little ones live for being the center of crowded birthday party festivities, whereas others (like Tess, also in Chapter 5) are slower to warm up, and still others would be happiest avoiding them altogether. The likelihood your child will melt down at a birthday party is highly related to where he falls along this continuum.

Filled with Temptations

Still, certain settings are universally notorious for eliciting tantrums, and they share some notable characteristics. In addition to being overstimulating and/or unfamiliar, these places are often rife with temptation. If you show me temptation, I'll show you a young child who will start to test limits. There are obvious temptations, such as the candy and toys found in stores, sometimes housed in their own separate aisles but often deliberately placed in unavoidable locations (by the checkout lines), as if marked with flashing neon signs commanding children: *Ask your parents if you can have me. If not, melt down **impressively and immediately.*** Then there are more subtle ones, not necessarily comprised of items your child wants to take home, but enticing enough to merit touching (bins of screws and bolts at home-improvement stores), petting (feather dusters in the cleaning supply aisle), or engaging with in some other (often inappropriate and typically highly time-consuming) fashion. A little girl I recently heard about wouldn't walk another step until she squeezed every single sponge in the bin at the drugstore. Why did squeezing the sponges hold such appeal?

Because many (although not all) young children thrive on sensory input—they love bright colors, things that are squishy, funny noises, sparkles. All they want to do is touch, play with, throw, or caress items that have these qualities. Parents, of course, respond to this behavior with variations on "no" or "stop that," which then leads to limit testing or defiance, which lands us squarely in the territory of—say it with me now!—tantrums.

> Surround a toddler with temptations and watch the limit testing begin.

And of course it's not just stores that are rife with temptation. Other people's homes can be equally enticing, given all that's new and unfamiliar, and those that are not childproofed (think: Thanksgiving at your great-aunt Martha's) can be particularly alluring, with their steep staircases, china cabinets, and other assorted novelties. Playgrounds with even just one piece of equipment geared to older kids (read: the forbidden fruit) can be a minefield, as can playdates or birthday parties where—for reasons I continually cannot fathom—there are treats or cake in plain view (and possibly within reach) that kids can't eat until they wait for the go-ahead.

Rules, Rules, and More Rules—or One Big (Impossible) One

Each of these situations highlights a third characteristic of those settings most likely to elicit tantrums, which is that is that they require children to follow many different rules, frequently at the same time. Maybe there's a lot of "stuff," or a lot of people, or a lot of standing still, or a lot of needing to move quickly—these settings are easy to recognize because they are essentially echo chambers for parents urging, "Watch out!" and "Stop!" and "This way!" and "I said over here!" and "Didn't I tell you to stay next to me?" and "Stop yelling!" and "The answer is no!" and "You're not being a very good listener!" and countless other toddler parent classics. Or, if there aren't a lot of rules, there is one *really* important one with high stakes for everyone ("No matter what you do, you absolutely cannot touch Aunt Martha's antique vase collection that is inexplicably exactly at your eye level even though she knows we come to Thanksgiving every year and that we haven't given you up for adoption"). When we place more demands on children than they may be able to handle at a given time, or put a great deal of pressure on one in particular, once again, we're stoking the coals for a tantrum in the not-very-distant future.

So the characteristics of settings that lead to tantrums tend to have a few things in common when we look at the world through our little one's eyes (as we are continually attempting to do, until it's almost a habit): they are overstimulating to the senses, they are packed with temptation, and they require a high level of compliance with rules. And what about when we look through our own eyes? Are there settings that are particularly tricky because of what *we* bring to the table as parents? Of course. As always, when it comes to the interactions around tantrums, more often than not, "it takes two."

How Some Places Set *You* Up to Melt Down— or at Least Get Stressed Out

Our kids are clearly more likely to have tantrums when they accompany us into settings that heighten our own stress and frustration levels and those that test our patience even on occasions when we enter them alone. Think no further than your local Department of Motor Vehicles. There is always at least one toddler throwing a tantrum when I go to the DMV. Is my DMV particularly overstimulating? Hardly. A den of temptation? Not so much, even by toddler standards. Are there rules to follow? Sure, but no more than there are in most places. Rather, I'd hypothesize, what makes the DMV particularly ripe for toddler tantrums is that, while there, parents more often than not experience feelings of frustration, impatience, and helplessness, all feelings that don't exactly lead to top-notch parenting. As highlighted in Chapter 4, if we're stressed and irritated to begin with, we're certainly going to be that way with our children, which then puts us squarely on the tantrum map.

Now, the DMV is so universally stressful that it's almost a parody of itself in that way. There are other settings, however, less obvious ones, that some parents may find particularly stressful for some reason or another. I have a client who is supersensitive to light and has learned that taking along her sunglasses wherever she goes is essential to decreasing her preschooler's tantrums, given how irritable and impatient *she* becomes when the environment is too bright for her. And if we get anxious in crowds or long lines—think airport security or holiday shopping—it may well be our own difficulty regulating our emotions that is driving the tantrum interaction. The key here is cultivating an awareness of the settings that make *you* crazy, so that you can preemptively build in

> Your child is ripe for a tantrum in the places that stress you out.

measures to calm yourself down, thereby decreasing the likelihood your child will melt down.

The other critical piece that parents bring to the table is the capacity for *shame*. This is a big one. I can't tell you how many times I've had moms and dads in my office bemoaning how "embarrassing" it was when their toddler had a tantrum at the supermarket, or how they "just wanted to disappear" when their little one melted down on the playground. And when parents feel embarrassed by, or ashamed of, their toddler's behavior, toddlers experience this as a real rupture in the connection. Think about it: if you are hyperfocused on what the mother over by the slide is thinking about your horror of a two-year-old, then you are 100% not in your two-year-old's corner—potentially right when she needs you there most. When we feel more allied with other observers or (as we perceive them to be in those moments) judges of our child's tantrum than we do with our child, our child no longer feels the emotional presence and connectedness that's so often key to his ability to calm down. "Of course he just started crying and yelling more," I'll frequently say—always empathically—to parents in my office. "In the moment you gave an unsure and apologetic smile to a stranger, you pretty much hung him out to dry." Our little ones pick up on it when we feel ashamed of them, or somehow puzzled and freaked out by their behavior. They become even further dysregulated, and meltdowns go from bad to worse.

> When your child starts to fuss, aligning yourself with adult onlookers instead of your kid robs him of the connection he needs to gather self-control and avoid melting down.

Shame is, of course, a natural human experience and one with deep roots. If it seems too narrow to consider it only in the context of tricky settings, think about how the same toddler or preschooler behavior can seem perfectly fine to you in some places but feel unacceptable in others. In broad strokes, we all know different behavioral expectations typically apply in a house of worship than at the playground, for example. But the line can be blurrier. Maybe it's OK for your three-year-old to make noise at your own house and most others—but not Grandma's. Whether you feel slightly chagrined when your expectations aren't met or your cheeks are blazing and you're hanging your head may depend on your individual background, personal experiences, and triggers. So again, self-awareness is key. Think about the factors likely to be most potent in setting off your shame reaction when your child begins to throw a tantrum, thereby rupturing your connection with your child and likely increasing the tantrum's intensity. Are you more likely to feel ashamed around strangers or people you know well? In a restaurant, store, library, or house of worship? Among family members or among friends? This is not an exhaustive list of questions, nor are the answers necessarily mutually exclusive. The point is to set your thoughts in motion so that you can begin to see more clearly what settings may be particularly difficult for *your* child given the baggage you *yourself* are carrying.

Clearly, there are a great many factors to consider when it comes to thinking about settings that will increase the likelihood—and subsequent duration and intensity—of our little ones' tantrums. Regardless of what makes a setting "tricky," however, and we've looked at both universal and more esoteric variables, there are some things you can do—before, during, and after—to make these experiences a bit easier to handle.

Q "It's never enough with my son. If I give him a special treat, he asks for another one and melts down when I say no. He has a million toys, but when his grandparents come to visit, he asks them—to their faces!—for a present and has a tantrum unless they happen to have one with them. How do I stop him from being so greedy? It's embarrassing!"

A Wow. There is so much in this question. First of all, let's put yourself in your son's place. He's a little kid, just learning about how the world works. So far, among many other things, he knows that he really digs special treats and really digs getting presents. Can you blame him? Those things are pretty great; I'm a big fan myself. He has also learned that asking for things sometimes gets you things (simple cause and effect), so he is giving that strategy a shot, with both you and your parents. He hasn't yet learned the manners behind when it's OK to ask and when it's not, as well as how to feel grateful for what he already has. Young children are often, by definition, hedonists: if something feels good, then they want more of it. It's that simple. This is normal, and does not represent greed or selfishness. If you want your child to begin to feel and experience gratitude (which has been linked to various positive outcomes, so I agree it's important), start by modeling what that looks like; as discussed in Chapter 8, modeling is the number-one way to teach children at this age, and this goes for overall values as well as more concrete behaviors. Try reading books about gratitude or just speaking aloud about things for which you're grateful (for example, "It's good to be home after a long day! I'm so grateful for our cozy home!").

Second, it sounds like your son's grandparents do sometimes have presents for him when they visit, and that therefore his query is sometimes rewarded. So long as a present is available *sometimes* when they come over, he is going to keep asking for one every time. This is because there are few things more powerful than intermittent reinforcement. And if you're trying to teach him not to ask for the present, but rather just to wait and stand by to see if they have one, this is a very tall order, and he may well not be able to comply with it given his excitement and impulsivity. In sum: if grandparents are sometimes bringing over presents and your son asks about this when they show up, cut him some slack.

Finally, it sounds to me like your own embarrassment over what you are perceiving as your son's greed is also playing a role here. My guess is that your disapproval of his behavior is influencing your reaction to his tantrums, which is likely in turn making them worse. When we prioritize a third party's reaction (a parent or in-law, a fellow parent at the playground, an onlooker in a public place) over our children's feelings at a given moment, our children sense that and can experience it as a rupture, which then makes the tantrum that much worse.

Before Arriving at the Tricky Setting

1. *Anticipate and assess.* As always, this is so key, particularly when it comes to thinking about or planning an outing day or weekend. Before you go somewhere, think about whether it might be a "tricky setting" according to the criteria set forth beginning on page 199. What will the experience be like for your child with regard to temptation level and sensory input? Will there be a lot of rules that she'll need to follow? Is this a setting that you yourself find difficult in some way or where you are apt to feel ashamed if your child does end up having a hard time? Remember from Chapter 2 that the chain of events and other factors leading to a tantrum offer multiple points of intervention or prevention. Anticipate these problems and you might be able to keep the chain from forming at all. Examples that frequently come up in my practice include (but are clearly not limited to) supermarkets, warehouse stores, drugstores, playgrounds, family gatherings, hotels, and public transportation (including airports).

2. *Be strategic about planning your days.* If you have a list of errands to do (and your child needs to accompany you), think about what time you need to start leaving the house (see Chapter 10 for more on this "activity"!), and make sure to allot more time than you need for the various transitions involved. Also consider the order in which you make your various stops and keep the number of things planned reasonable. Think about when your child is going to nap (if he still does) and when and how you are going to build in a meal and/or snacks. As a general rule, it's best not to hit tricky settings when you, your child, or both of you are already worn out; exhaustion makes most things more difficult, and tricky settings are no exception. It can be tempting to structure your various stops according to geography, which is how we grown-ups tend to plan things; in this case, though, it may make sense to think about the order in terms of the "tricky quotient" for your little one. Certainly, I don't recommend crisscrossing town several times in an afternoon, but looking at characteristics other than geographical location may ultimately benefit the interactions you have with your child and lead everyone to have a better day.

3. *Don't squeeze in that one last thing—especially if said thing involves a tricky setting.* I don't care how badly you need new lightbulbs. Your family will function better by candlelight than you will if you schlep your toddler or preschooler to the drugstore right before dinner after a packed afternoon. It's better to cut something off your to-do list for the day than it is to try to do too much and inevitably wind up having a nightmare "last stop," which will then set the tone for the evening, often one of the most difficult times of the day to begin with (again, see Chapter 10). You can always order lightbulbs online, which leads me to:

4. *Modern technology for the win.* If you live in an area where it's possible, and it's a financially feasible option for your family, don't be afraid to make life easier by relying on the wonders of the Internet. For example, if your child is a nightmare in supermarkets and drugstores, think about whether it makes sense to avoid the challenge altogether by using an online grocery delivery service. I don't recommend you do this every time; we can't model (and therefore teach) that avoidance is always possible or preferable. We raise resilient children with good coping skills in large part by letting them have experiences that may be frustrating or overwhelming and by showing them that they can get through it, in part with our support. As usual, there's no formula that dictates when to allow and when to preempt our children's frustration; it's a question that necessitates your taking into account many other variables. As an example, if you barely slept,

your child had an overstimulating playdate that morning, and you've been generally stressed about your child's eating of late, I'd recommend ordering groceries online. Alternatively, when you have a leisurely afternoon ahead, everyone's cheery, and you don't need too many things, a trip to the supermarket may be just the fun outing you're looking for.

5. *Set the scene for your child (and maybe build in a reward).* Remember the importance of structure and of having clear and well-defined expectations (as emphasized in Chapter 7)? This idea applies here as well. Tell your child where you are going and what she can expect. What will the place look like? Who will be there? Will it be crowded? What are you going to do there? About how long will it

> Toddlers and preschoolers need practice in handling challenging settings—but not on days when you're both already stressed out.

take? What—and this part is key—do you need from her? Do you need her to hold your hand or to stay next to you? What about using an inside voice—is that important? Is there something that might be particularly challenging (a toy or bakery aisle, Aunt Martha's vase collection)? If you're going to a store, it can be extremely helpful to discuss beforehand whether your child will be allowed to get anything and, if so, what kind of thing. If the answer is definitively yes or no, then say that and stick to it. If it depends on her behavior, then be clear about that too; it's OK to build a reward into an outing, so long as the expectations around it are clear: "If you stay next to me and use your inside voice the whole time we're at the supermarket, you can pick out a treat on our way out. If I need to give you more than two warnings, though, we won't be able to do that." Having a brief, casual conversation about all of this *in advance* will help buffer the overstimulation, anxiety, and limit testing that often leads to meltdowns. Here, the distinction between a reward and a bribe is important. A reward is promised in advance, before the possible negative behavior and limit setting begins; this way, you are not unintentionally reinforcing that behavior. A bribe, on the other hand, occurs once the unwanted behavior (in this case, a tantrum) has begun, and therefore sends the message that yelling/screaming/crying can be effective in getting the thing you want.

> Remember: rewards are promised in advance; bribes are offered once a meltdown has begun and reinforce that behavior.

6. *Become a team with your child.* This piece is so, so important; your child does best when he feels like you "get" him (see Chapter 6), and this is doubly true in tricky settings. Your child needs to know that you're there for him, in his corner rooting for his success, rather than just waiting for the proverbial s#% to hit the fan. If he has the sense that you're somehow on different sides, with opposing goals, or that you're exasperated or nervous before you've even gotten started, the chances of a tantrum increase significantly. This point comes up again and again and again in this book because its importance cannot be emphasized enough. When you communicate, even if only nonverbally, feelings of stress, overwhelm, or powerlessness over the situation at hand, your child picks up on this and starts to feel the same way, which may well manifest in a tantrum. One way to help ensure that you approach the tricky setting as a team is to give the task at hand a name that evokes fun and positivity, such as Mommy and Aaron's Adventure in Costco, Jonas's Journey to the Supermarket, or The Smiths Take On Thanksgiving. Incorporate words like "journey," "adventure," "fun, " and "exciting" to conjure up good associations. "Super-duper" is also always a winner. Feel free to really get into it—come up with a song or cheer you can sing as you go.

> Naming your outings in a way that makes them seem like parent–child adventures encourages collaboration and connection.

7. *Come prepared.* What does your child need to succeed? Snacks? Something to play with? We can't predict what's to come, but we can prepare for it.

8. *Regulate yourself.* The few seconds before entering a tricky setting with your child are essential for doing whatever it is you do to make sure you feel as calm as possible. Remember: you are the thermostat, not the thermometer. Take a deep breath, close your eyes for two seconds, and picture your "happy place," hum a few bars of a current favorite tune—it doesn't matter what you do, so long as you do something to bolster yourself with the calm confidence you'll need to set the tone for success.

While at the Tricky Setting

Now you're there. You've done all the prep work, and you find yourself in a setting that you know is filled with invisible tantrum fairies, all conniving to ensure that your child completely loses her mind before you leave. Here are some strategies to employ to counter their covert efforts.

1. *Engage your child.* Sounds simple, because it is, at least in theory. A tricky setting is a great place to talk to your little one about his interests (with how you do so, of course, depending on his expressive/receptive language skills). Ask him to tell you his favorite joke again, or about the episode of *Paw Patrol* he watched over the weekend, or about what he wants to be for Halloween. Beware asking questions based on *your* interests, or that are vague in nature (such as what he's doing in preschool these days), as they will likely yield a string of "I don't know" or yes/no answers or blank stares, none of which will serve the purpose of actually engaging him and may even further your own frustration (and therefore be counterproductive to the larger purpose at hand: tantrum avoidance). Sometimes young children feel pressured by questions in general and respond better to statements. I recently started a conversation with Henry by letting him know that I was having trouble choosing my favorite song from *Moana*, because it's a toss-up between "You're Welcome" and "Shiny." He responded by telling me about his own song preferences, something I don't think he ever would have done (or at least not right then) if I'd asked directly.

> Toddlers and preschoolers like to be asked about their interests just as adults do.

2. *Play a game.* If a regular old conversation won't cut it, play a game with your child as a diverting activity. Depending on his age, he may be able to name all the words he can that rhyme with "feet" or give you opposites for words you provide. He may be into guessing what kind of animal makes a particular sound or naming as many colors as he can. "I Spy" is also a good one for tricky settings; so is naming everything you see of a particular color. The idea is to keep your child engaged and having fun so that he can avoid the pitfalls of the tricky setting (overstimulation, temptation, testing limits), thus defying the tantrum odds.

3. *Use strategic attention.* Instead of tossing a "don't" at your child every few seconds for the thing(s) she's doing wrong, start off by thanking her for the things she's doing right, or just saying something nice (details on using this strategy are in Chapter 8). "Look how you are keeping your hands down at your sides!" or "It's so great that you're using your inside voice," or "I really love spending time with you and holding your hand" (this last

example having the added benefit of drawing attention to the connection between you).

4. *Sing a song together.* Self-explanatory. The longer, the better. You knew there had to be a reason someone wrote "The Wheels on the Bus," didn't you?

5. *Race.* I've already recommended this distraction, and it can work beautifully in some settings. Obviously you may not be able to have an all-out running race in every place, but young children love racing in any form. Try "I bet you can't WALK to the oranges over there before I count to five." Or sometimes young kids just love the word "race" and are even happy to do so while simultaneously holding your hand, despite that not making any sense to anyone who understands what a race is. Just go with it. Oh, and along the same lines, I feel like I shouldn't have to say this, but please just let it go if they cheat (read: "I want to start over here," and "here" is 10 feet ahead of you). In this moment, our goal is to prevent a tantrum, not to be Captain Fairness (thereby potentially causing a tantrum, in a complete plot reversal). I actually saw this happen the other day. Eye on the ball, people.

> When it comes to positive engagement of your toddler, don't be a stickler—"sense" and "rules" are not the point here.

6. *"I bet," in general.* I wrote the preceding tip and then realized that the phrase "I bet" merited its own bullet point. Toddlers and preschoolers go nuts when you "bet" they can't do something; they rise to the challenge almost every time. To name a mere five out of countless possible examples a weary parent might use in a tricky setting:

"I bet you can't do the hokey pokey all the way down this aisle. No way!"

"I bet you don't know what color this is" (pointing to some object or other).

"I bet you can't count everything we have in our cart so far."

"I bet you can't name everyone in this room."

"I bet I can't close my eyes and *not hear* you while you X." (If this phrasing sounds random and a bit awkward, it's because I happened upon it by accident with my own little guys, but it has been a hands-down winner and thus merits sharing.)

7. *Give your child jobs.* To the extent your child views herself as your helper—and ideally really embraces the role—she most likely won't have a tantrum. This is something you can set up in advance and then make good on once you're there. If in a store, have your child help you get things off the shelf, put things in your cart, place items into a bag, and so on. If at a family gathering, have your child help you carry things in or remind you to tell a particular story to a particular person there. If no immediate jobs come to mind, make one up. I am not above asking Henry to "help" me figure out how many hair elastics I have in my bag.

8. *Reflect feelings.* It stinks to be in front of a whole lot of tempting objects and not be able to get one. It really, really does. Let your child know that you get this and that you don't take for granted, say, that he walked down the cookie aisle in the supermarket without falling apart, or that he stayed away from Aunt Martha's vases for the second year running.

9. *Modulate your voice* when it comes to the demands you're placing on your little one. Sometimes, in tricky settings, your child does something really annoying. Other times, your child does something that could be dangerous. Make sure your reaction, and the tone of your voice, reflects the difference, so that your child isn't experiencing nonstop commands and criticism from the word "go."

> Constant commands and criticism are a surefire way to trigger a tantrum in a tricky setting.

10. *Continue to be a team with your child.* Invoke the clever name you came up with for the errand/outing, and/or your cheer or song, often. Let your child know, verbally or with your smiles and body language, that you enjoy spending time with her. This is particularly important if your child is starting to engage in behaviors that you find slightly—or more than slightly—embarrassing or shameful. Please note my phrasing there: "that *you find*" and *not* "that *are*." Little ones become overstimulated and tend to test limits in tricky settings because they are little, *not* because they are bad. The elderly woman who just "tsk-tsked" and admonished you with her eyes either does not know or does not remember that. *You* do. Your toddler or preschooler needs you to join with him, to signal, somehow, that you know how hard his little brain is working to keep it together, that you have his back. What he does not need—and

what will undoubtedly make his behavior worse—is for you to throw him under the bus, instead joining the elderly woman, rolling your eyes along with her in solidarity.

11. *Practice ongoing self-regulation.* The deep breath you took before you entered the tricky setting? Repeat that every couple of minutes. Pretend you're on a warm beach in the Caribbean, feeling the tropical breeze through the palm trees rather than the sharp chill of the frozen foods aisle. Keep coming back to making sure that you are calm, particularly if you feel like your toddler or preschooler may be on the verge of falling apart. Which leads me to, last but not least:

12. *Don't push it (a.k.a. Cut your losses if you need to).* That is: leaving is an option. If you've accomplished even a fair amount of what you set out to, and it feels like you're starting to be on thin ice with regard to your toddler's ability to hold it together, it's OK to abandon ship. Even on Thanksgiving. If you do leave before you intended, either before or during a meltdown, this is *not* a failure—either on your part or on that of your little one. Tricky settings are hard; they (read: I) don't call them "tricky" for nothing. You might implement all of the strategies in this chapter to a tee, and yet your child still falls apart. This is because he's a child. You may lose your patience. This is because you're a parent. Children and parents aren't perfect, and there's nothing like a tricky setting to make that abundantly clear.

After Leaving the Tricky Setting

1. *Pat yourself, and your little one, on the back.* Really. You (both) did it. No matter how it went. If it didn't go as well as you might have hoped, take the opportunity to repair and reflect (see Chapter 6, and page 167 in Chapter 8). Think about what you might do differently next time—without beating yourself up—and do something to reestablish the connection between you and your child.

2. *Make good on any rewards you may have promised your child* (presuming she held up her end of the bargain).

3. *Exhale.*

12

"A Tantrum Is Quite Possibly the Last Thing I Need Right Now"

How to Reduce Tantrums under Difficult Circumstances, from Travel to Moving to Divorce

Just as young children tend to throw more tantrums at certain times of the day and in particular types of settings, so too are there situations or circumstances that lend themselves to an uptick in the frequency and/or severity of tantrum episodes and interactions. As a general rule of thumb, any circumstance in which toddlers and preschoolers are likely to feel powerful emotions is one in which their parents are likely to see more frequent and intense meltdowns than usual. This knowledge is powerful; to the extent you can predict when your child is apt to "have all the feels," you can anticipate the possibility (or probability) of tantrums and adjust your parenting game accordingly. Of course, sometimes it's easier to make this prediction than others, which is why I divide tricky situations into two different categories, those you can anticipate and those you cannot.

Before we start with the former, I want to make one more point about "tricky situations" in general. That is, they're tricky for a reason, and not just for kids. Just as thinking about how we feel in a crowded shopping mall can help inform our understanding of how young children likely feel in the same setting, so too can we look at our own responses to the situations discussed in this chapter as windows into how our little ones may react, both emotionally and behaviorally. The circumstances described in this chapter—ranging from a child's feeling sick to moving to introducing a new baby—can be, and often are, enormously loaded for parents. It's important, therefore, whenever you are faced with a "tricky situation," not only to look to the pointers in this chapter, but also to refer back to the points raised in Chapter 4—that is, to be cognizant of what you, as a parent, are bringing to the table and, more precisely, the tantrum interactions. Always important? Absolutely. Even more so when in or approaching so-called tricky situations? Yes and yes and yes.

Tricky Situations We (Parents) Can Predict

I can't emphasize enough that the ability to anticipate tantrums is one of the most effective tools you have at your disposal. The more preparation you can do as parents, the less likely your child is to be overwhelmed by big feelings, because there's a critical difference between *having* big feelings and being completely *blindsided* by them. The best place to start is with a quick assessment of the current state of love and limits in your home:

- Are you feeling connected to your child, having more positive than negative interactions on the whole?
- Are stable routines and structures in place?

If the answer to either of these questions is no, that's where your efforts need to focus. Look back to Chapters 6 and 7 for ideas of how to build up both love and limits if or when one of them seems as though it may be lacking. In ordinary daily life with a toddler or preschooler, it's natural for these variables to ebb and flow a bit. Most of the time, there's no need to pay attention to the small peaks and valleys, and they may not even be noticeable. When tricky situations lie ahead, however, really looking closely at the presence, and levels, of love and limits in your home becomes increasingly important. After all, it is your child's relationship with you and general feeling of safety/security that will allow him or her to experience strong emotions without feeling overwhelmed by them. And less overwhelm = fewer tantrums.

In the name of decreasing overwhelm, please do your child (and yourself) a favor and avoid adding unnecessary stress during the times described on the following pages. Do not start potty training your toddler a month before his baby sister is due. Do not transition your child out of her crib the week after she was home with the flu. Do not take away your child's pacifier right before you move to the suburbs. You get the idea. Just as it's a terrible idea to cut out carbs the day after you've been fired, it's unproductive (and also insensitive) to take away your child's trusty comforts—be they diapers, a crib, or a pacifier—during these potentially overwhelming times.

Let's go through some common predictable tricky situations:

Travel

Whether by plane, train, or automobile, on trips ranging from two days to two weeks, young children may be apt to have a tough time (read: throw more or worse tantrums). Traveling, by definition, means a complete change in surroundings, often from the familiar to the (at least relatively) unfamiliar. There may or may not be a time change (and time changes alone are often sufficient to throw a whole family system out of whack), and parents frequently experience a kind of low-level yet pervasive nervousness for the duration. They're either "on guard" for unpredictable travel incidents or worried about how various aspects of the trip will play out. Will the hotel mattress be decent? Will my mother-in-law have her usual unrealistic expectations about how my kids should behave? For all of these (among other) reasons, young children can experience travel and time away from home as disorienting or even upsetting. *You* know that making sure you have everyone's boarding passes is more important than digging a granola bar out of your bag, but, from your toddler's perspective, you're just distracted, exasperated, and way less responsive to his snacking needs than usual. As with everything, there are vast individual differences here, and yet I have found that even the most adventuresome, flexible little ones often have more tantrums during and in the wake of time away. How to handle this?

1. Before you leave, let your child know what to expect, what's going to happen when. Maybe even make a simple picture book with drawings or photos (nothing fancy!) that maps this out day by day.

2. Similarly, review social and behavioral expectations in advance, as specifically as possible:

> "The house we are renting will have a pool. It is very important that you not go near the pool unless a grown-up is there."

> "Aunt Doris will ask you for a hug. It is OK not to hug her if you don't want to. Let's talk about what you can say or do instead."

3. To the extent possible, bring your child's usual schedule and routines into the different setting. Can you get him the same breakfast cereal

to eat in the morning? Bring her own sheet to put on the mattress? (Along the same lines, consider adding a white noise machine and paper blackout shades to your packing list!) Still FaceTime the grandparents on Sunday? Read some of the same books at bedtime? (Books are heavy to pack, but lugging a few favorites is 100% worth it so that you can replicate the bedtime routine you do at home as closely as possible.)

4. On the flip side, embrace the change—we call vacations "getaways" for a reason. Help your kids enjoy the change in your daily routine. Point out the different kinds of flowers and trees that don't grow where you live. Giggle about Grandpa's photos of you at prom. And be gentle with yourself about "slippage"—your child may have more screen time or sugar than she'd have at home, and that's OK.

5. Be conscious of how you schedule and spend your days. If this sounds a bit vague, it's because I can't provide a formula; it all depends on your family's preferences. Some children and families do better with more activity and less unstructured time. Other children and families do better with more downtime and fewer set plans. The point is to be thoughtful about how you balance both activity/structure and downtime, and to consider not only your own but also your children's needs in this regard.

6. Remember to connect to your children consciously and intentionally. Again, while you're keeping track of logistics and making plans so that the time away is a success, your little one may be experiencing you as distracted, nervous, exasperated, or all three. *Anticipate* this (there's that word again!), and make sure to find time to devote yourself fully to your child, doing whatever it is that she wants to do. If that's stare at the lizard on the wall for what seems like an inordinately long period of time, then so it goes (our family just went on a tropical vacation, and this was a favorite pastime of my boys).

7. After your return, it's likely your child will be exhausted, both physically and emotionally. This is key to remember not only in the hours immediately after you get home, but also in the days (and sometimes even weeks) that follow, when parents often see an increase in tantrums. Be understanding and compassionate about this, bringing on the hugs and cuddles, while also prioritizing getting back into typical routines as quickly and seamlessly as possible. Let your child know that you get it: "Going away and then coming home again is *exhausting*, right?" If his or her emotions continue to seem all over the place following time away, consider making a book about the trip, or just spending some time describing the various

events in order of how they unfolded. You can highlight fun memories and look at the pictures you took. In so doing, you are helping your child organize his or her experiences, which little brains can't always do by themselves at this stage.

Your Child Is Sick

First, a caveat: when I say "sick" here, I mean with the typical cold/cough/fever that so often plagues young children, particularly during the winter. Having your child diagnosed with more debilitating/serious conditions presents a unique set of circumstances (for various reasons) that merits a more in-depth treatment than can be given in this context. Although we can't literally predict with any accuracy the exact moment when a virus is going to strike our little ones, we can prepare for this kind of sickness more generally, which is why I'm including this scenario as a predictable tricky situation. When toddlers and preschoolers feel sick, they often feel emotionally overwhelmed as well. Why? Because feeling sick *stinks*. And it's unfamiliar, and maybe scary, and generally just the *worst* (can you tell I'm not such a great patient myself?). Much like travel, children's illnesses often take a toll for way longer than parents expect; the physical symptoms may be long gone, but the emotional hangover—which can very often be increased tantrum frequency or severity—lingers on.

When young children have a perpetually runny nose or hacking cough, they rarely complain about it. They don't tell you that the pressure in their sinuses builds every time they lie down, or that there's a sharp pain in the back of their throat every time they swallow. Young children lack both the expressive language and conceptual knowledge to be able to share such information. So what do they do instead? Show you how they feel through their behavior. If your child's tantrums have become more frequent or intense in the context of more coughing or congestion than usual, chances are good the two are related. So what to do?

1. Many of the strategies presented in Chapter 8 apply here. In particular:

Zero In on Your Toddler's Emotions (page 154). When your little one is sick, chances are she's telling you how lousy it is with some combination of bodily fluids and crankiness. As a parent, one of the most powerful things you can do during these periods is label and reflect the accompanying emotions. Empathize with how much it can stink to be sick, with both your words and facial expressions/body language; beyond this, though, tell your child stories about how you feel when you're sick or how you felt when you were a kid. Maybe you feel frustrated because you can't run around like usual, or maybe you remember how disappointed you were when you had to miss your best friend's birthday party in second grade. There are some great children's books to read when toddlers and preschoolers are sick that facilitate these conversations (we love *Llama Llama Home with Mama* in our house).

Tap the Power of Distraction (page 158). Children feel better physically—as do we all—when they're distracted. Although some may disagree on this, my feeling is that when little ones are sick in bed, rules about screen time get lifted, as (developmentally appropriate) TV shows, movies, and videos are incredibly powerful tools for distracting young minds. Of course, children also love being read to, listening to music, and playing low-energy games when they're not feeling well. Sometimes parents worry about the extent to which they may be forming bad habits when they take this path: "Won't Emily start to think she can watch this much TV all the time?" In my experience, no. Despite not having a sophisticated understanding of what being sick is, young children do get that their typical day doesn't involve lying in bed all day long and that certain things are different on sick days. Also, remember, we don't parent well when we let our fear of our children's emotional reactions dictate the choices we make. If Emily, once healthy again, were to continue to expect to watch the same amount of TV, you'd simply correct her, at which point she might get upset, and *both she and you could handle it.*

2. Think: sleep. It's always important, of course, but sleep becomes even more critical when your toddler or preschooler is under the weather. Ensuring that your child is getting all the sleep he or she needs to land back in good health is paramount, which means you may need to be a bit more of a stickler about bedtime, perhaps even pushing it earlier than usual. This is not something you need to explain, or even say out loud, to your child; chances are you can move bedtime up by 10 or 15 minutes (often all it takes) without your child's even noticing (thereby bypassing a possible power struggle).

3. A quick note on medicine. Many parents struggle with kids who run away shrieking and crying at the mere mention of this word (here's looking at you, Henry). Keep in mind that medications indicated solely for

pain management (such as acetaminophen) are distinct from those necessary for a full recovery (at times antibiotics, for example); the extent to which you want, or need, your child's compliance may vary accordingly. I recommend actively collaborating with your pediatrician (ideally, someone you both trust and respect) so that the rules made around compliance are in keeping with medical necessity. Once medical necessity is established, to my mind, physical health comes first. This is a subtle way of suggesting, as I have to many clients, that this may be a time for bribery (two chocolate chips for every milliliter ingested), or a chocolate milkshake (into which the medicine is blended). If that doesn't do it, talk to your pediatrician about what else you can try.

You're Moving

The facts of this particular tricky situation don't need a great deal of explanation: you live in one place, and soon you'll be moving all your stuff and living in another place. Just as moves are disorienting (overwhelming emotion alert!) for adults, so too are they for young children, although there are—as always—individual differences here, as well as important factors to consider related to the move itself. If your family is moving to a new apartment down the hall from your current place, that is likely less disruptive than moving to a whole new neighborhood, or from the city to the country (or vice versa), or to a different state or even country.

1. Be thoughtful and intentional about how and when you tell your child about an upcoming move; ideally, wait for at least some of the details (logistical plans, moving date) to be worked out so that you can provide as much concrete information as possible. As we know, young children are concerned about the world primarily insofar as it relates to them directly (egocentrism!), so present the information accordingly. What is going to be the same for your child—same bed, same preschool, same stuffed animals? What is going to be different—different bedroom, different bathroom, different walk/drive to preschool?

2. Connect with your child by giving him space to feel all his (possible) feelings about the move, and not just the "good" ones. When parents frame an upcoming change as the best or most exciting thing in the world without allowing a child to feel ambivalent or even completely differently, we see an increase in tantrums, in part because there's a rupture in the parent–child connection. Is moving exciting and fun? Sure, it can be. It can

also be sad, annoying, and (almost always) exhausting. This is a situation in which it can be very helpful for parents to model what it's like to have two (or more) feelings at once: "I'm excited to move into our new house because I love the pantry there—it's so big and can hold so many snacks! I'm a little nervous, though, because so many things will be new. I'm also sad to leave the bathtub in this house because it's so big." By saying things like this, you're opening the door for your child to do the same. She may then tell you what she's excited, nervous, and sad about. Or she may say she's just excited, in which case there's certainly no need to push your child to have complicated or multiple feelings. And, of course, a two-year-old may just look at you and repeat "house." Even here, though, you're still modeling emotional fluency, which is key as children learn language.

3. Making, and then reading together, a book about the move, so that a child can view the event as part of a larger narrative rather than an isolated, random event, can be very nurturing; include pictures of the old place and new place and mention the various feelings that may arise.

4. Rituals can also be nurturing to children and, in a sense, add structure to experiences that may be emotionally overwhelming. For example, going around to each room in your old house, naming a fun/nice/important thing that happened there, and even saying "thank you" can help children say good-bye to a home. Similarly, going around to each room in your new house, saying hello, and introducing yourselves can be a fun and meaningful way to get started in a new home. Be creative and embrace the silly!

5. Adherence to normal and stable routines is critical in the days, weeks, and months following a move. Children feel *contained* when bedtime looks the same in the new house as it did in the old house, when the contents of their snack shelf remain the same, when their bath toys accompany them to their new bathroom. For the same reason, be consistent about behavioral expectations. Allow your child to see that, although the physical structure of your home may be different, the structures that exist within it remain the same. Of course, there may be routines you can't replicate, or new ones that have to be established. Perhaps you used to walk to preschool and now you need to drive. Or you lived in a climate where your child barely needed a jacket, and now she has to bundle up. In these cases, be sensitive to the fact that it may take time for your child to get used to the change and even say that out loud (for example, "In Florida, we didn't need jackets, and here we do. That's a big change! It's gonna take some time to get used to"). Your naming the experience will be comforting to your child

and help decrease any overwhelming feelings. You might even make a list of things that are different in the new house and things that are the same, or a book that lays this out in pictures.

Your Child Is Getting a New Sibling

Perhaps the most famous, or infamous, predictable tricky situation of all is the new baby. In many cases, the new baby arrives after Mommy is pregnant for nine (except in real life it's actually 10) months, although the situation clearly looks different when siblings are adopted or carried by a surrogate. Regardless of how your child's sibling is going to enter the world and your family, my strong bias is that your child needs to know that this is coming down the pike as soon as it's a done deal. There are other early childhood experts—for whom I have great respect—who disagree with me on this point, noting that it's not beneficial emotionally for young children to know about a new sibling too far in advance. Although it's important to consider the needs and characteristics of individual families, I have never seen a toddler or preschooler who didn't know—on some level—that something was afoot from the very early stages. Maybe Mommy is tired all the time, or maybe she's throwing up. Maybe Daddy is just acting differently in some way, or parents are speaking more in hushed tones, or going into other rooms to take phone calls.

I've said it many times, and I'll say it once more: *young children pick up on your energy*. When there is a shift in energy that is unacknowledged or unexplained, this is not a comfortable feeling for little ones and can result in behavior/mood changes and, yes, tantrums. I can't tell you the number of times I've seen a toddler's tantrums improve once parents share with them the upcoming change that is going to occur within their family. Recently I met for the first time with a couple, Chris and Marta, who came in reporting that their three-year-old daughter, Nadia, had been having fairly intense daily meltdowns for the past month or so. I asked whether this might be in response to Mom's pregnancy; Marta was visibly pregnant and had confirmed that she was about 21 weeks along. Both Chris and Marta immediately answered in the negative; Nadia's tantrums couldn't possibly be about her future baby brother, they assured me, as they hadn't yet told her she would be getting one. It seems they had read that telling her too soon would "just make her nervous." I asked Marta whether she was still picking Nadia up and carrying her. "No," Marta replied. "We told her that the doctor said I couldn't do that anymore. She seemed fine with it."

"Except she's not fine," I responded. "She's expressing pretty big and unmanageable emotions at least once a day." I went on to explain that, regardless of whether Nadia understood her mother was pregnant, she undoubtedly knew something was up—not only because of how her mother clearly looked and was acting, but also because now a mysterious "doctor" had been invoked. When young children hear "doctor," they think "sick," and so it was possible, even plausible, that Nadia believed there was something wrong with her mother, something way scarier than having a baby in her tummy. And yet she had also taken her parents' cue, as young kids often do, that this was not a topic open for discussion. Nadia's intense tantrums, I hypothesized, likely stemmed from this double dose of anxiety. To help Chris and Marta see this, I imagined what Nadia would say if she could put her feelings into words: "I don't understand what's going on with my mommy. I think she might be really sick, because the doctor told her she's not allowed to pick me up anymore. Or maybe she just doesn't want to pick me up anymore. I can't ask what's going on because Mommy and Daddy don't want to talk to me about it. I'm scared and I feel alone."

My sense, I told Chris and Marta, was that Nadia's tantrums would vastly subside if her parents clued her in to what was going on, using simple and loving language. I encouraged them to show her pictures of her brother from the ultrasound and to read books about getting a new baby brother. I gave Marta a script: "Because your baby brother is growing in my tummy, I can't pick up things that are heavy because I could hurt myself. [Don't, I advised, say that you could hurt the baby, lest Nadia interpret that as your somehow choosing her brother over her.] I really miss picking you up, though! And I'm *mad* that the doctor said that, even though I know I have to listen! You're heavy because you're such a big girl, and you're also my special baby and always will be. Let's make sure we snuggle together more, now that I can't lift you up anymore."

I made sure to provide reassurance to both Chris and Marta—as I often do—that no, they had not damaged their daughter for life and that, more than anything else, this was an opportunity for a substantial and meaningful repair. Sure enough, when Chris and Marta returned for a follow-up session two weeks later, they reported that Nadia's meltdowns had ceased almost immediately after she learned about her baby-brother-to-be.

Needless to say, much has been written about how to ease young children's transitions to older-sibling-hood. Here are merely a few quick pointers:

1. Both before and after the baby (or child) joins your family, implement regular "special time" with your (first) child every single day, even

if only for five minutes (for how to do this, see the end of Chapter 6). Your child needs to be able to *count on* feeling the connection between you to feel anchored and safe during an otherwise emotionally tumultuous period. When you have your first baby, everyone says to "sleep when the baby sleeps." Regardless of how useful you found this guidance then (and I certainly didn't, mostly because of LAUNDRY), it no longer applies. Now, when the baby sleeps, your priority is to seek out your toddler or preschooler, push through the exhaustion, and connect. In the moment, this may not be what you feel like doing (cue feelings of resentment, followed by guilt), but I promise it will be worthwhile given the positive impact on your child's emotional adjustment.

2. During this special time (or other, nonplanned moments in which you find yourself without the baby), say out loud how nice it is not to have the baby around (despite how much you adore the new cuddlebug in town) and that a part of you really misses the time when it was just you and your older child. I remember a few months after Zeke's birth, I invited Henry to come with me into the drugstore to pick up a prescription while my mom stayed with Zeke in the car outside. Would it have been easier to have left them both in the car? Of course. The ease of my day is inversely correlated to the number of times I need to interface with car seats. And yet I knew that even three minutes of special Mommy–Henry time (even on line at the drugstore) would be meaningful—to both of us. As we waited for the pharmacist to come to the counter, I looked at Henry and held up my hand. "High five," I said. "Zekey's not here." Henry's face lit up as he jumped up to slap my hand with his. By giving voice to these sentiments, I was showing him that all of his feelings about Zeke were OK and understandable. Much like moving (and most big life changes), having a new baby sister or brother is not exclusively fun and exciting, and can also be extraordinarily difficult. Interestingly, and no doubt related, when we got back to the car, Henry asked me to lift him up so he could give Zeke a kiss. It was as if, by getting permission to enjoy Zeke's absence for a few moments, his heart could then open up to his baby brother in a pure and authentic way.

3. If your four-year-old expresses anger toward his or her baby sibling, remember the distinction between feelings and behavior: "Feeling mad that Baby Gregory is using your old baby swing is completely OK, sweetie; trying to pull him out of it is not." Give her alternatives; instead of hitting little Greg, she can hit one of her stuffed animals, or draw a picture about how mad she is, or squeeze up her face really tight.

4. *To the extent possible* (italicized because there is likely a limit to this, and no one—child or parent—benefits if you make yourself crazy), keep your child's daily routines intact and predictable. So much else is topsy-turvy, so your child will rely more than usual on familiar structures.

5. Be gentle on yourself. Call in supports. Get help during tricky times of day (bath and bedtime, anyone?). Order takeout. Get things delivered. These may be obvious points (which is why I'm keeping it brief), but please, please keep them in mind. Your older child needs *you* to feel less overwhelmed during this crazy time. You know what doesn't need you? The laundry. The groceries. To the extent your financial and logistical circumstances allow, figure out ways to get out of non-child-related tasks and activities.

You Are Separating from Your Partner

Needless to say, just as there are myriad different kinds of parenting partnerships, there are countless types of separations, all of which involve different and complicated dynamics. Others have written extensively and expertly about how to help young children cope with their parents' separation and/ or divorce (see the Resources section), and, so as not to do the issue a disservice (or to stray too far from the subject of tantrums), I am merely going to touch upon it here. These types of family changes are monumental for young children and therefore, of course, often lead to increased tantrum frequency and intensity. Here are just a few general pointers related to what I have found to be some of the most common dynamics and scenarios:

1. Remember the importance of consistency with regard to limits. If your child is alternating between the care of two parents, either in the same or different homes, this can be somewhat destabilizing. The way to address this is to ensure that daily routines and behavioral expectations remain as similar, and thus reliable, as possible. Some parents want to be the "fun one," or for their home to be "the one that feels like a treat," and this temptation is normal. It's also more about the parent than the child. What's actually best for kids is that both parents, and both home environments, uphold consistent structures that keep them feeling safe and secure.

2. Be thoughtful about the transition between parents or homes. Much like leaving the house (see Chapter 10), this transition is an activity unto itself, and so needs to be afforded a great deal of care and intentionality.

Having a regular calm and connected ritual for how you do this—both saying good-bye to one parent and saying hello to another—can do much to calm young children's understandably overwhelming emotions during these times. I worked with a mother who made sure to always have the same snack (I want to say vanilla wafers and grapes) ready for her son when his father would drop him back at her apartment after the weekend. The two of them would sit on the couch as he munched, while she read him three different storybooks that she picked out from his shelf in advance. Being able to predict, and even picture, this weekly ritual did much—for both mom and son—to ease this otherwise emotionally charged time.

3. Keep in mind that if your toddler or preschooler is having more or more intense tantrums than usual in the context of a separation, this is not your partner's fault. Or maybe it is, frankly. Maybe your partner wanted the divorce and you didn't, or your partner cheated on you and left you no choice but to leave, or . . . whatever. The point is, whether or not you blame your partner, the rage you feel toward him or her will not help your child to feel less overwhelmed. Find other outlets for your emotions—your therapist, your best friend, the punching bag you just ordered online—so that you can show up for your child in a calm and regulated state.

4. Finally, build in opportunities for your toddler or preschooler to assert some control over a situation that no doubt feels (and is) completely out of his or her control. For example, if your child is going to have a new room in a new space, give him some power over decorating it. Let him pick out his comforter, or rug, or a pirate ship tent for the middle of the room. If your child will be going between homes, let her choose two different bags or suitcases, one that you pack and one that she does.

Tricky Situations We (Parents) Cannot Predict

Family transitions make for a great segue into the second category of tricky situations: those we can't predict. Although we typically know when a new sibling or a separation is coming down the pike, there are a host of other family circumstances about which we don't have the same lead time. A grandparent or other family member becomes ill and passes away. Someone gets into an accident. A nanny doesn't show up one day and disappears. Our partner leaves us without warning. We need to put down a beloved pet. These situations vary, of course, in their traumatic impact, but they have in common their unpredictability. Life can, after all, change on the turn of a dime, and although thankfully it generally doesn't, this chapter wouldn't be complete without some mention of these scenarios.

When it comes to many of the circumstances I just named, the word "tricky" is euphemistic and could even, in some cases and depending on contextual details, be replaced by "traumatic." As stated up front, this book is not about those tantrums that toddlers and preschoolers have as a trauma reaction, which are best addressed with professional guidance (see page 236 for how to find a professional to work with your family, should this apply). Unpredictable situations are not, however, always traumatic, and despite not having the luxury of lead time to prepare, there are still measures parents can take to minimize their little ones' emotional overwhelm, thereby decreasing the likelihood of an increase in tantrums. As always, love and limits are the things that will get you through, and they're never more important than as an anchor during the crises and upheavals that occur. Managing your children's potentially overwhelming emotions will hinge on their knowing both that you still *get* them and that you've still *got* them—no matter what else is going on around you.

This is good news. Because when life gets unpredictable, or tricky, or traumatic, we, as parents, become even more imperfect than usual at handling our little ones' tantrums. We don't take good care of ourselves, so we're more likely to snap, or get triggered, or take things out on our kids that the sane and stable part of us knows aren't their fault. These are times when we need to make a point of going back to basics, back to the themes you've found woven throughout this chapter and the book as a whole.

Q "My mother just got diagnosed with breast cancer. I'm so scared and upset, and also so distracted. My four-year-old daughter clearly knows something is wrong, but I don't know how to explain it to her."

A Replace "breast cancer" in this question with any type of medical diagnosis, or even just awful news in general, and this is a very common question (sadly, it's a somewhat common question without replacing those words as well). Something happens that makes you more emotional than usual—be it sad, angry, anxious, upset—and you don't know how much to share with your little one. Although these situations can look different, I tend to offer three guiding principles that go hand in hand: First, be honest. Your child already knows something is up and will only be soothed by having this reality acknowledged aloud. Second, be developmentally appropriate and focus on your child's experience of what's going on, as this is the piece that's important to her. Do not get bogged down in surrounding details that are irrelevant (at least to her). Third, let your child know that there are grown-ups helping so that she doesn't attempt to take on this responsibility, which can be harmful on numerous levels. So, how would these principles look when applied to this question? Perhaps like this:

- Honest: "I am feeling sad this week. I found out that Grandma has something bad in her body." [Beware of the word "sick," as your child may come to fear his or your "sickness" (that is, a virus or a cold) as something very sad or scary.]
    - Not: "I'm fine! Nothing's wrong! I just have something caught in my eye!"
    - Not: "I found out that your grandmother was diagnosed with a rare form of breast cancer."
- Developmentally appropriate and focused on your child's experience: "You may find it harder than usual to get my attention."
    - Not: "I'm hanging on by a thread and barely keeping it together."
    - Not: "My relationship with Grandma is complicated, and so a lot of feelings are coming up for me, and I'm also grappling with existential thoughts about my own mortality."
- There are grown-ups helping: "Grandma is meeting with doctors who will help her body get better. I am talking to Daddy, and Uncle Max, and some of my grown-up friends so that I can feel less sad. That is not your job."

Of course, this conversation would vary depending on your child's age, and it's impossible for me to provide every permutation or a script for the different ways the conversation might continue. As a general rule, though, the principles described are a good way to structure difficult conversations with young children, thereby decreasing their—and your own—anxiety. And, of course, it's always nice to close with some variation of "I love you so much, and we are all going to get through this." Because you do, and you are. Whatever it ends up looking like, you are.

A few weeks ago, Henry refused to get out of the car. I'm grateful to say that the week hadn't been a traumatizing one for our family, but it hadn't been an easy one either. Our regular babysitter had quit unexpectedly, my father-in-law's Parkinson's had taken a turn for the worse, and Zeke had gotten in the habit of waking up between 4:50 and 5:10 A.M.—and not going back to sleep. Anyway, it was about 5:30 P.M.; I had just gotten the boys home from day care/preschool, and it was about nine (yes, you read that correctly, NINE) degrees outside. I got Zeke out of his car seat first, then walked around the back of the car to get Henry out. I somehow managed to get him unbuckled despite holding all 30 pounds of Zeke, who would not let me put him down. The second Henry was free, he darted to the front seat, where he stayed put and refused to budge.

I was freezing. Zeke was heavy. His nose was dripping snot onto my new winter jacket (no big deal, but also: new jacket). I was exhausted. I halfheartedly attempted a few tried-and-true strategies with Henry—Could he get out of the car without my hearing him if I closed my eyes? Could he beat me to the top of our front stairs?—then started to lose my temper a bit, because (to run it down for you again): tough week, 30 pounds, arctic temperatures, snot. Henry glared at me and declared, "Mommy, you are *embarrassing* me!" I should note, just in case it needs clarification, that Zeke and I were the only other people in the driveway, and I can say with confidence that neither of us was doing anything remotely embarrassing. At this point, I realized three fundamental truths at the exact same time (any *Hamilton* fans among you?):

1. I felt like throttling my child. He clearly had no idea what "embarrassing" meant, and I had the urge to tease him—nah-nah style—about that. I genuinely felt all intellectually superior—*to my own three-year-old son.*

2. I flashed forward to Henry's teenage years, when no doubt I'll hear these exact words said in a more appropriate, if also wounding, context.

3. I recognized that Henry was experimenting with language, using an expression he had clearly heard someone else say (a friend in his class, it turned out, when I queried later) in an effort to convey how steaming mad he was at me.

And so I took a deep breath and empathized with what I knew Henry *meant*: "Wow, honey. I can see that. You do *not* want to get out of the car.

You are really *angry*, huh?" At which point he looked at me, smiled, got out of the car, and gave me a hug. After all, as you may recall from the Introduction, I am an early childhood psychologist and the author of this book, no less; I've got these situations nailed. Except what actually happened was that Henry looked at me, shrieked something unintelligible (I want to say he also bared his teeth, wild animal style, but that part's fuzzy), and stayed exactly where he was.

Spoiler alert: I don't remember exactly how I got Henry—or, more accurately, how Henry decided to get—out of the car that night. There wasn't really any magical moment to speak of. I do remember that he didn't really cheer up until after dinner and that by bedtime Zeke's runny nose had become a full-fledged cold. The operative word in that last sentence, though, is "bedtime"; we made it through the day that day, just as we do every day. And the thing that helped most—also the part I remember most vividly—is the pause I was able to put between Henry's declaration of embarrassment and my own reaction. In that brief moment, I could simultaneously get a clear glimpse into my own emotional state (irrational rage) *and* ask myself what was going on for Henry. Once I posed that question to myself—not even consciously—I was able to see that, like a lot of almost-four-year-olds, he was playing around with language and attempting to assert his autonomy by separating himself from me. I could then respond to him in a present and connected way.

Of course, it helped that I had just met with a father who relayed a similar tale of his daughter's telling him he was "gross" every time she didn't want to do something. "Q-TIP," I had reminded that dad, whose feelings about his own history of being teased as a kid for being overweight had clearly been triggered by his daughter's apparent insult. "Quit taking it personally. Acknowledge the feeling behind the word, so that your daughter knows you understand what she means, which is not, of course, that you're gross (a word she has likely just learned and is experimenting with), but rather that she's mad and doesn't want to listen to you. You can have a conversation about manners in another, less heated, moment." Having this exchange so fresh in my mind helped me follow my own advice. Which is the same thing that I hope having the stories in this book fresh in your mind will do for you.

When we can pause to ask ourselves what's really going on in a given interaction with our little ones—with regard to their stage of development, our own emotional reactions, and the surrounding circumstances—we can often stave off a meltdown, or at least prevent one from worsening. In so doing, can we create magic? No. OK, well, maybe occasionally. What about just make it easier to get through the day, so that we can enjoy those bed-time snuggles in a real and present way? Yes. To this one, a solid yes. Plus, the more we practice, the more prepared we are for the long parenting jour-ney ahead. If we can begin to recognize our children's tantrums as both a normal part of their development and just one piece of a larger interper-sonal context, we'll be that much more skilled at doing the same when the eye rolls, annoyed sighs, and sarcastic retorts of the tween and teenage years come at us at warp speed. Although the behaviors may look different as they grow, our children's expressions of emotion and need for autonomy are going to be around for the long haul.

If we're lucky.

Resources

Parenting Toddlers and Preschoolers

Organizations

Aha! Parenting: *www.ahaparenting.com*
American Academy of Pediatrics: *www.aap.org/en-us/Pages/Default.aspx*
American Psychological Association: *www.apa.org/index.aspx*
Center on the Developing Child (Harvard): *https://developingchild.harvard.edu*
Child Mind Institute: *https://childmind.org*
Essential Parenting: *http://essentialparenting.com* (particularly the "Practices"
    section: *http://essentialparenting.com/resources/practices*)
Hand in Hand: *www.handinhandparenting.org*
Happily Family: *www.happilyfamily.com*
Zero to Three: *www.zerotothree.org*

Australian Pediatric Society: *www.auspaediatrics.com.au*
Australian Psychological Society: *www.psychology.org.au*
British Psychological Society: *www.bps.org.uk*
Canadian Paediatric Society: *www.cps.ca*
Canadian Psychological Association: *www.cpa.ca*
Irish Paediatric Association: *www.irishpaediatricassociation.ie*
Royal College of Paediatrics and Child Health: *www.rcpch.ac.uk*

Attachment

Center for Attachment Research: *www.attachmentresearch.com*
International Attachment Network: *http://ian-attachment.org.uk*

Trauma

National Child Traumatic Stress Network: *http://nctsn.org*
Somatic Experiencing Trauma Institute: *http://traumahealing.org*

Books

Attachment

Cassidy, J., & Shaver, P. R. (Eds.). (2016). *Handbook of attachment: Theory, research, and clinical applications* (3rd ed.). New York: Guilford Press.
  - Unquestionably dense, intense, and intended for professionals, but for the ambitious, this volume really does cover it all.
Gopnik, A. (2017). *The gardener and the carpenter: What the new science of child development tells us about the relationship between parents and children.* New York: Picador.
  - The author of the seminal *The Scientist in the Crib* uses developmental psychology research to show how important it is that kids be raised to be kids, in all their messiness and unpredictability.
Hoffman, K., Cooper, G., & Powell, B. (2017). *Raising a secure child: How Circle of Security parenting can help you nurture your child's attachment, emotional resilience, and freedom to explore.* New York: Guilford Press.
  - The best and most practical guide, in my opinion, to all that we know about parent–child attachment, why it's important, and what we can do day to day to use this knowledge as we raise our little ones.
Why attachment parenting is not the same as secure attachment, by Diana Divecha (2018, *Greater Good Magazine*)
  https://greatergood.berkeley.edu/article/item/why_attachment_parenting_is_not_the_same_as_secure_attachment
  - I know this is not a book, but the amazing Diana Divecha has written the article I've wanted to see for years (and didn't get around to writing myself)—one that spells out the important distinction between "attachment parenting" and "creating a secure attachment." Despite the misleading use of the same term, these two ideas are *not* the same thing, and, sadly, the resulting confusion has led many parents to feel completely unnecessary guilt and distress. Honestly, I put this article in the "important public service announcements for parents of young children" category.

Building on Brain Development

Brazelton, T. B., & Sparrow, J. D. (2006). *Touchpoints—Birth to three* (rev. ed.). New York: Da Capo Lifelong Books.

- This, along with the sequel, *Touchpoints—Three to Six,* is kind of a bible of child development, written from the joint perspectives (read: knowledge, wisdom, insights) of a renowned pediatrician and psychiatrist. Both can be read cover to cover or used as references when needed (the second part of both books is organized alphabetically by topic).

Lieberman, A. F. (2017). *The emotional life of the toddler* (updated ed.). New York: Simon & Schuster.

- The best book I've found on really getting inside a toddler's mind from a social-emotional standpoint.

Plooij, F. X., van d Rijt, H., & Plas-Plooij, X. (2017). *The wonder weeks: How to stimulate your baby's mental development and help him turn his 10 predictable, great, fussy phases into magical leaps forward* (5th ed.). Arnhem, The Netherlands: Kiddy World Publishing.

- A week-by-week guide to your baby's first 20 months, with a focus on what's going on in your child's mind that likely leads to fluctuations in the "3 C's" (crankiness, clinginess, crying). So helpful!

Siegel, D. J., & Bryson, T. P. (2012). *The whole-brain child: 12 revolutionary strategies to nurture your child's developing mind.* New York: Bantam.

- An excellent description of how children's brains are wired, with effective ways to apply this science to everyday parenting issues.

Sunderland, M. (2016). *The science of parenting* (2nd ed.). London: Dorling Kindersley.

- Another book with practical advice for parents based on brain science, with color pictures and many "key points"—like a textbook that's not actually a textbook.

Communication and Discipline

Faber, A., & Mazlish, E. (2012). *How to talk so kids will listen and listen so kids will talk* (rev. ed.). New York: Scribner.

- Incredibly concrete and practical tips for doing just what the title says. Written in a highly accessible—and funny!—style.

Kazdin, A. E., & Rotella, C. (2014). *The everyday parenting toolkit: The Kazdin method for easy, step-by-step, lasting change for you and your child.* Boston: Mariner Books.

- More on the workings of the "ABCs" of children's behavior from one of the top behavioral researchers in the field of child psychology.

Lansbury, J. (2014). *No bad kids: Toddler discipline without shame.* CreateSpace Independent Publishing Platform.

- A collection of articles by an author with a unique ability to see the world through toddler eyes and to write about "respectful parenting practices" that benefit parents and kids alike in concrete, "real-life" terms.

Markham, L. (2012). *Peaceful parent, happy kids: How to stop yelling and start connecting.* New York: Perigee.
- A great book with the important premise that an emotional connection between parent and child is fundamental to enjoyable—and easier!—parenting.

Siegel, D. J., & Hartzell, M. (2013). *Parenting from the inside out: How a deeper self-understanding can help you raise children who thrive* (10th anniversary ed.). New York: TarcherPerigee.
- A wonderful exploration of how parents' histories and emotions influence the ways in which they interact with their children.

Family Dynamics

Cummings, E. M., & Davies, P. T. (2011). *Marital conflict and children: An emotional security perspective.* New York: Guilford Press.
- A super-thorough and insightful look at how marital/partner dynamics influence child development, particularly from an emotional/psychological standpoint.

Faber, A., & Mazlish, E. (2012). *Siblings without rivalry: How to help your children live together so you can live too.* New York: Norton.
- An easy-to-read "bible" of sorts on issues to consider when raising more than one child, including useful comics (really!) and poignant reflections from a group of adults who wish their own parents had done things differently in this area.

Feeding/Eating

Of all the books on feeding young children, these are my favorite, along with the materials found on the author's website: *http://ellynsatterinstitute.org.* The focus is on practical ways to encourage our little ones to have a *good relationship with food*—everything else (physical health, etc.) flows from that.

Satter, E. (2000). *Child of mine: Feeding with love and good sense* (rev. ed.). Boulder, CO: Bull Publishing.

Satter, E. (2008). *Secrets of feeding a healthy family: How to eat, how to raise good eaters, how to cook* (2nd ed.). Madison, WI: Kelcy Press.

Sleep

These books represent different approaches to sleep, sleep learning, and sleep training. Sleeping issues are very personal; if you need help in this area, I encourage you to look at a few in order to choose the method that seems best for you, your child, and your family.

Henry, E. (2016). *The compassionate sleep solution: Calming the cry.* CreateSpace Independent Publishing Platform.

Kennedy, J. K. (2015). *The good sleeper: The essential guide to sleep for your baby—and you.* New York: Holt Paperbacks.

Pantley, E. (2016). *The no-cry sleep solution for newborns: Amazing sleep from day one—for baby and you.* New York: McGraw-Hill Education.

Weissbluth, M. (2015). *Healthy sleep habits, happy child: A step-by-step program for a good night's sleep* (4th ed.). New York: Ballantine Books.

Articles/Websites

These articles/websites are ones I return to again and again in my practice, continually emailing them out to the families with whom I work. (Yes, there are many, so I cherry-picked just a few of my favorites.)

Don't carpe diem, by Glennon Doyle Melton (2012, *Huffington Post*)
    www.huffingtonpost.com/glennon-melton/dont-carpe-diem_b_1206346.html
The cries that bind: Connecting with children emotionally, from Hand in Hand Parenting
    www.handinhandparenting.org/article/the-cries-that-bind-connecting-with-children
6 things the happiest families all have in common, by Eric Barker (2014, *The Week*)
    http://m.theweek.com/articles/444395/6-things-happiest-families-all-have-common
Why I yelled at my son (who didn't deserve it) (2018, *Fatherly*)
    www.fatherly.com/love-money/relationships/father-and-child-relationships/why-i-yelled-at-my-son-who-didnt-deserve-it
    • Part of a great series *Fatherly* does called "Why I Yelled." Real stories about real dads with real tempers. While we're at it, both Fatherly.com and Motherly.com have some very good content if you take the time to pore through (or sign up to receive their emails).
Mindfulness for Children, guide from the *New York Times* (2017)
    www.nytimes.com/guides/well/mindfulness-for-children
    • Basic tips for children of all ages, as well as activities that promote empathy and compassion, as well as focus and curiosity.
Dr. CBT Mom
    www.drcbtmom.com/blog
    • Wonderful writing by Dr. Ilyse Dobrow DiMarco, another mom and psychologist, about some of the most common struggles that accompany motherhood.
Meghan Leahy, parent coach
    www.mlparentcoach.com
    • Meghan Leahy is the parenting expert for the *Washington Post* and is very much worth checking out!

Parenting and Family section (*Greater Good Magazine*)
    https://greatergood.berkeley.edu/parenting_family
- Published by the Greater Good Science Center at the University of California–Berkeley, the "Parenting and Family" section of *Greater Good Magazine* is filled with accessible articles that translate the latest research on a range of useful topics into layperson language. Search for topics such as self-compassion, cultivating gratitude, the role of technology, and so forth.

Getting Professional Help

Division 53 of the American Psychological Association, the Society of Clinical Child and Adolescent Psychology, offers a directory of child therapists in the United States and Canada who practice using evidence-based treatments and techniques: *https://sccap53.org/find-a-therapist*.

Also through the Society of Clinical Child and Adolescent Psychology, this website provides information about a range of evidence-based child therapy approaches, as well as tips for choosing a therapist: *http:// effectivechildtherapy.org*.

Evidence-Based Therapies That Focus on the Parent–Child Relationship

Child–parent psychotherapy
Circle of Security
Parent–child interaction therapy
Parent management training
The Incredible Years

Evidence-Based Therapies for Couples

Emotion-focused therapy
Gottman method therapy

Resources for Toddlers and Preschoolers
(and Slightly Older Kids Too)

Increasing Emotional Fluency

Books

Bang, M. (2004). *When Sophie gets angry—really, really angry*. New York: Scholastic Paperbacks.
- Such a great portrayal of what makes a little girl get *really, really* mad and what she does in response. Her experience is treated with respect, as nothing more or less than what it is: human.

Best Behavior series: *www.freespirit.com/series/best-behavior*
- With simple words and great pictures, these books are very helpful when it comes to targeting specific negative behaviors and replacing them with more prosocial ones. Titles are great and straightforward—*Hands Are Not for Hitting, Feet Are Not for Kicking, Teeth Are Not for Biting*—and many are available in board-book form for the really little ones, as well as longer, more in-depth paperbacks.

Cook, J., & DuFalla, A. (2015). *But it's not my fault! (Responsible me!)*. Boys Town, NE: Boys Town Press.
- A humorous book in verse that chronicles the school-day misadventures of Noodle, a little guy who keeps getting into trouble and has a hard time taking responsibility for his own behavior. A list of good tips for parents/educators at the end.

Cornwall, G. (2017). *Jabari jumps*. Somerville, MA: Candlewick.
- A sweet story about a little boy who overcomes his fear of jumping off the diving board with the help of his patient, loving father.

Dewdney, A. *Llama* series: *http://llamallamabook.com*
- Join little Llama as he experiences adventures, emotions, and challenges that look remarkably like those facing your own child.

Holmes, M. M., Mudlaff, S. J., & Pillo, C. (2000). *A terrible thing happened*. Washington, DC: Magination Press.
- More of a straight-up bibliotherapy book (that is, a book used within therapy contexts), but still so good, about a little boy who sees something terrible (we never find out what) that makes him anxious and angry and gets help from a counselor: "Sometimes parents help children figure out their feelings. Sometimes teachers or other grown-ups help. That is how Sherman met Ms. Maple."

Karst, P., & Stevenson, G. (2000). *The invisible string*. Camarillo, CA: Devorss.
- A great book for young children experiencing loneliness or separation anxiety, about how people who love each other have hearts that are always connected by "an invisible string" of love.

Levis, C. (2012). *Stuck with the blooz.* Boston: HMH Books for Young Readers.
- A wonderful, imaginative children's book about how sometimes the best way to feel better is to make space for our difficult feelings.

Parr, T. (2005). *The feelings book.* New York: LB Kids.
- No one does feelings better—in the most vibrant colors and cutest drawings—than Todd Parr (see his website too: *toddparr.com*).

Rubinstein, L. (2013). *Visiting feelings.* Washington, DC: Magination Press.
- Colorful pictures and language help foster young children's awareness of their emotional states.

Saltzberg, B. (2010). *Beautiful oops!* (Illust. ed.). New York: Workman.
- For the child who's having a tough time understanding that it's OK (and natural, expected, even wonderful) to make mistakes.

Snel, E. (2013). *Sitting still like a frog: Mindfulness exercises for kids (and their parents).* Boulder, CO: Shambhala.
- A great introduction to mindfulness meditation, which has been shown to help children (and grown-ups too) learn to calm down, manage big feelings, and be more aware/patient overall. Comes with the added bonus of a 60-minute audio CD of guided practices.

Yamada, K., & Besom, M. (2017). *What do you do with a problem?* Seattle, WA: Compendium.
- A poetic book about how avoiding problems tends to make them worse and more difficult emotionally. If you face a problem head on, not only do you feel better, but you get to see what's hidden inside: an opportunity. *What Do You Do with a Chance?,* by the same authors, is also great.

Yolen, J., & Teague, M. (2013). *How do dinosaurs say I'M MAD?* New York: Blue Sky Press.
- Fun rhyming text about what the members of little kids' favorite species do when they're angry. Easy to read, concrete, and relatable. Part of the "How Do Dinosaurs . . . ?" series, which I recommend across the board.

Viorst, J. (2008). *Alexander and the terrible, horrible, no good, very bad day.* New York: Scholastic Book Clubs. (Original work published 1987)
- Because sometimes it's all just because we're having a bad day. Even for kids.

Viorst, J., & Blackall, S. (2014). *And two boys booed.* New York: Farrar, Straus and Giroux (BYR).
- A little boy (whose voice is *so* real) is nervous to sing in his talent show. Two boys boo. Our little boy makes it through. Because that's kind of how life goes. Such a great depiction (versus description) of emotions with a few fun lift-the-flaps to boot.

Magination Press: *www.apa.org/pubs/magination/index.aspx*
- Books designed to help children deal with a variety of common challenges and problems experienced by those 4–18, from the routine (school,

typical childhood fears, siblings) to the more difficult, such as illness, death in the family, and divorce. Written by mental health professionals and those in related child care professions. Particularly helpful are the Notes to Parents, which offer tips on using the books for parents and professionals.

Books That Heal Kids: *http://booksthathealkids.blogspot.com*
- A blog/compilation of book reviews by an elementary school counselor.

Videos/Articles/Websites

Daniel Tiger's Neighborhood (assorted episodes): *http://pbskids.org/daniel/videos*
- A PBS series inspired by *Mister Rogers' Neighborhood,* in which Daniel, a four-year-old tiger, experiences a range of unfamiliar and at times confusing social and emotional situations. The episodes include characters that young children love, as well as catchy tunes that get stuck in their heads (and yours).

GoZen!: *www.gozen.com*
- A series of animated videos that help children learn skills for resilience and general well-being. Also a terrific blog with entries by the wonderful Renee Jain, such as "A Mindful Minute: 3 Fun Mindfulness Exercises For Kids": *http://gozen.com/a-mindful-minute-3-fun-mindfulness-exercises-for-kids*

Sesame Street: Common and Colbie Caillat—"Belly Breathe" with Elmo: *www.youtube.com/watch?v=_mZbzDOpylA*
- A catchy, great tune with concrete pointers for how to "belly breathe" when you need to "chill your inner monster out."

Sesame Street: Dave Matthews and Grover Sing about Feelings: *www.youtube.com/watch?v=Po5lHYJJQfw*
- Poignant chords and amazing lyrics about how hard it can be to find words for what we are feeling.

Sesame Street: Lena Headey Helps Murray Relax: *www.youtube.com/watch?v=8ppOup8fp4E&index=3&list=PLBxHL1WwIyb9Ff1jqEWT8_TSQOmIy0ZMH*
- Murray was supposed to define "relax" for us viewers, but he panics when he forgets his lines. Lena Headey not only helps him remember, but shows him how to calm down by breathing.

Sesame Street: Me Want It (But Me Wait): *www.youtube.com/watch?v=9PnbKL3wuH4&index=1&t=8s&list=PLBxHL1WwIyb-uQLTm5B_Kk2mZ-SxYLAsF*
- Who knew Cookie Monster knew so much about strategies for waiting and self-control?

Create your own book for your child's experience: *www.twigtale.com/books*
- Whether you're embarking on a parents-only vacation, or you're moving, or you're ready to tackle potty training, Twigtale offers wonderful templates for creating narratives (and inserting your own photographs!) that help your child understand.

Divorce

Books

Brown, M., & Brown, L. K. (1986). *Dinosaurs divorce: A guide for changing families*. New York: Little Brown Books for Young Readers.

Higginbotham, A. (2015). *Divorce is the worst (ordinary terrible things)*. New York: Feminist Press at CUNY.

Levins, S., & Langdo, B. (2005). *Was it the chocolate pudding?: A story for little kids about divorce*. Washington, DC: Magination Press.

Masurel, C. (2003). *Two homes*. Somerville, MA: Candlewick.

Videos/Articles/Websites

Sesame Street Toolkit: Divorce: *www.sesamestreet.org/toolkits/divorce*

Death/Grief

Books

Buscaglia, L. (1982). *The fall of Freddie the leaf: A story of life for all ages*. West Deptford Township, NJ: Slack Inc.

Edwards, A., Ponciano, L., & Horwitz, J. (2014). *The elephant in the room: A children's book for grief and loss*. CreateSpace Independent Publishing Platform.

Higginbotham, A. (2015). *Death is stupid (ordinary terrible things)*. New York: Feminist Press at CUNY.

Levis, C. (2016). *Ida always*. New York: Atheneum Books for Young Readers.

Mellonie, B., & Ingpen, R. (1983). *Lifetimes: The beautiful way to explain death to children*. New York: Bantam.

Olivieri, L. (2007). *Where are you? A child's book about loss*. Lulu.com.

Parr, T. (2015). *The goodbye book*. New York: Little Brown Books for Young Readers.

Wilhelm, H. (1988). *I'll always love you*. New York: Dragonfly Books.

Videos/Articles/Websites

Growth from Grief: Moving Families Forward: *http://growthfromgrief.org*

National Alliance for Grieving Children: *https://childrengrieve.org*

NIH Clinical Center Patient Education Materials: Talking to Children about Death: *https://clinicalcenter.nih.gov/ccc/patient_education/pepubs/childdeath.pdf*

Sesame Street Toolkit: Grief: *www.sesamestreet.org/toolkits/grief*

Index

Note. *f* or *n* following a page number indicates a figure or note.

"ABCs" of tantrums, 17–22
Acceptance
    safety and, 123
    secure attachment and, 117–120
Activity level, 93. *See also* Temperament
Adaptability, 93, 130–131. *See also*
        Temperament
Age for tantrums. *See also* Developmental
        processes
    brain development and processes and,
        43–48
    normalcy of tantrums and, 29–31
    overview, 3–4
Aggression towards people or things, 15
Anger
    avoiding emotions, 173
    emotional reactivity of parents and, 86–90
    new baby in the family and, 222
    overview, 26–27
    strategies for dealing with tantrums and,
        157–158, 164
Antecedents. *See also* Triggers for tantrums
    "ABCs" of tantrums, 17–22
    behavioral chain analysis and, 32–33, 34*f*
    multiple factors and, 32–33, 34*f*
    overview, 32–33, 42
Anticipation
    settings for tantrums and, 204
    travel and, 215
Apologizing
    strategies for dealing with tantrums and,
        147–148
    after the tantrum, 167
Appreciation, 48–49

Approach/withdrawal, 93–94. *See also*
        Temperament
Arguing in front of children, 101–102
Assessing a situation, 204
Assessment, 15–17
Assumptions regarding tantrums, 8–9
Attachment, 116–120, 231, 232. *See also*
        Parent–child relationship
Attachment theory, 76
Attention
    giving children credit, 154
    leaving the house routines and, 189
    morning routines and, 185
    settings for tantrums and, 208–209
    strategies for dealing with tantrums and,
        149–153
Attention seeking, 38–39
Autonomy. *See also* Control
    expectations and, 72
    need for, 4
    overview, 58–61
Avoidance, 173

Bath time routines, 192–194
Bedtime routines, 180–181, 194–197. *See also*
        Sleep patterns
Behavioral chain analysis, 33, 34*f*
Behaviors
    "ABCs" of tantrums, 17–22
    emotions involved in tantrums and,
        26–29
    involved in tantrums, 24–29
    language delays and, 36–37

241

Behaviors (*continued*)
    modeling of, 145–147
    strategies for dealing with tantrums,
        164
    strategies that don't work, 174–175
Belonging, sense of, 93
Birthday parties, 199
Body image
    mealtime routines and, 190, 191
    personal histories of parents and, 82
Boundaries, 131–133
Brain development and processes. *See also*
        Developmental processes
    appreciating mental efforts of child,
        48–49
    emotionality and, 56
    impulsivity and, 50
    meeting children where they are, 63–66
    overview, 43–48
    resources regarding, 232–233
Breaking objects, 17
Breathing exercises, 195. *See also* Mindfulness
        skills
Brushing teeth
    emotionality and, 56–57
    morning routines and, 183
By-the-way factors, 102–105

Calling the police, threats of, 177
Calmness
    creating structure and routine and,
        137–138
    settings for tantrums and, 211
    strategies for dealing with tantrums and,
        165
Caregiver and child special time
    new baby in the family and, 221–222
    reconnection and, 122
Caregivers. *See* Parents
Causes of tantrums. *See also* Triggers for
        tantrums
    behavioral chain analysis and, 32–33, 34*f*
    list of possible causes to consider, 33,
        35–40
    multiple factors and, 32–33, 34*f*
    overview, 23–24, 30–42, 34*f*
Ceremonies, 53–55
Characteristics that fuel tantrums. *See also*
        Child
    egocentrism, 49, 61–63
    emotionality, 49, 56–58
    goodness of fit and, 92–97
    impulsivity, 49, 50–53
    meeting children where they are, 63–66
    need for control, 49, 58–61
    overview, 49
    rigidity, 49, 53–55
    strategies for dealing with tantrums and,
        142
Check-ins, 136–137

Cheerleading
    settings for tantrums and, 207
    strategies for dealing with tantrums and,
        152–153
Child. *See also* Characteristics that fuel
        tantrums; Parent–child relationship
    age for tantrums, 3–4
    goodness of fit and, 92–97
    resources for, 237–240
Choices
    morning routines and, 185
    strategies for dealing with tantrums and,
        161–162
Clarity, 137
Clothing, 72–73
Cognitive empathy, 62–63. *See also* Empathy
Communication
    addressing illness in a developmentally
        appropriate way, 226
    emotionality and, 58
    invalidation and, 170–172
    keeping it short, 156–157
    resources regarding, 233–234
    settings for tantrums and, 207
    strategies for dealing with tantrums and,
        156–157
Compassion, 108
Connection. *See also* Parent–child
        relationship
    being present and listening during a
        tantrum, 163–166
    creating structure and routine and, 138
    fear of parents and, 109–111
    foundation of, 113–116
    moving and, 218–219
    overview, 112
    parent–child relationship and, 118–120
    reconnection, 120–122
    repairing and reflecting after a tantrum
        and, 167–168
    safety and, 122–123
    strategies for dealing with tantrums and,
        158
    travel and, 215
    tricky situations and, 213
Consequences, 17–22, 180–181
Context of the tantrum, 5–6, 17–22, 42. *See
        also* Triggers for tantrums
Control. *See also* Autonomy; Characteristics
        that fuel tantrums
    bath time routines and, 193
    example of, 60–61
    expectations and, 71–72
    meeting children where they are, 63–66
    normalcy of tantrums and, 8–9
    overview, 49, 58–61
    rituals and, 54
    separation of parents and, 224
Coping skills
    self-injury and, 15–16
    validation of emotions and, 41

Correlation, 31–32
Creativity, 140–141
Cultural factors, 75

Daddy and child special time
new baby in the family and, 221–222
reconnection and, 122
Daily routines. *See* Routines
Dawdling, 57
Day care, 136
Death, 240
Deescalating tantrums
"L words" and, 105–111
roles of parents in, 69–70
strategies for dealing with tantrums and,
    163–166
Department of motor vehicles (DMV),
    201–202
Desserts, 191. *See also* Eating patterns
Destroying objects, 17
Developmental processes. *See also* Age for
    tantrums; Brain development and
    processes; Normalcy of tantrums
addressing illness in a developmentally
    appropriate way, 226
attachment and, 76
expectations and, 71, 73
meeting children where they are, 63–66
normalcy of tantrums and, 29–31
personal histories of parents and, 83
phases and, 96–97
theory of mind and, 65–66
Dialectical behavior therapy, 33*n*
Disappointment, 173
Discipline. *See also* Parenting practices
good cop/bad cop and, 100–101
"L words" and, 105–111
overview, 6–7
personal histories of parents and, 78–80
resources regarding, 233–234
safety and, 125–129
strategies that don't work and, 180–181
Distractibility, 93. *See also* Temperament
Distraction
morning routines and, 185
sickness and, 217
strategies for dealing with tantrums and,
    158–161
Divorce of parents, 223–224, 240
DMV trips, 201–202
"Doorknob comments," 102–105
Dressing, 72–73
Duration of tantrums, 16, 61–63

Eating patterns
mealtime routines, 189–192
morning routines and, 183
personal histories of parents and, 82
as a possible cause, 33, 35

resources regarding, 234
snacking and, 192
Effectiveness of tantrums, 37–39
Egocentrism. *See also* Characteristics that fuel
    tantrums
example of, 60–61
expectations and, 71
meeting children where they are, 63–66
overview, 49, 60, 61–63
Emotional awareness, 47–48
Emotional contagion, 62–63. *See also*
    Empathy
Emotional empathy, 62–63. *See also* Empathy
Emotional regulation. *See also* Emotionality;
    Self-control
brain development and processes and,
    47–48
goodness of fit and, 93
of parents, 86–90
resources regarding, 237–239
settings for tantrums and, 207, 211
strategies for dealing with tantrums and,
    144–149
Emotionality. *See also* Characteristics that
    fuel tantrums; Emotional regulation;
    Emotions involved in tantrums; Feeling
    brain
avoiding emotions, 173
example of, 60–61
expectations and, 72
meeting children where they are, 63–66
new baby in the family and, 220–221
overview, 49, 56–58
of parents, 86–90, 174–175
predictability and, 129
resources regarding, 237–239
sickness and, 216–217
strategies for dealing with tantrums and,
    144–149, 154–158, 164
strategies that don't work and, 170–172,
    174–175
telling a child how to feel, 172–173
travel and, 215–216
Emotions involved in tantrums. *See also*
    Emotionality; Labeling feelings
appreciating mental efforts of child, 48–49
brain development and processes and,
    45–46
overview, 26–29
time-outs and, 107
validation of emotions and, 39–41
Empathy
bedtime routines and, 196
being present and listening during a
    tantrum, 163–166
egocentrism and, 62–63
responding to tantrums and, 108
sickness and, 216–217
situations we can't predict and, 227–228
strategies for dealing with tantrums and,
    142–144, 157–158

Energy levels, 184
Engagement, 208
Environmental factors, 35–36, 102–105, 198–204. *See also* Settings for tantrums
Events. *See also* Tricky situations
    as a possible cause, 35–36
    that we can predict, 213–224
    by-the-way factors and, 102–105
Executive functioning skills
    impulsivity and, 50
    leaving the house routines and, 186–187
    overview, 46–47
Exhaustion, 83–86
Expectations
    behavior and, 30
    creating structure and routine and, 135–136
    leaving the house routines and, 186
    mealtime routines and, 189–190
    meeting children where they are and, 63–66
    moving and, 219–220
    overview, 70–73
    personal histories of parents, 74–83
    settings for tantrums and, 200–201, 202–203, 206
    strategies that don't work and, 177–178
    structure and, 131–132
    travel and, 214
Explanations, short, 156–157
Expressive language skills, 36–37, 47. *See also* Language development
Extinction burst, 133

"False belief" tasks, 65
Family factors. *See also* Home environment; Parents
    new baby in the family, 220–223
    overview, 91–92
    resources regarding, 234
    role of, 97–102
    separation of parents and, 223–224
    by-the-way factors and, 102–105
Family meetings, 136–137
Fear, 109–111
Feeding problems. *See* Eating patterns; Hunger
Feeling brain, 45–46, 56. *See also* Brain development and processes; Emotionality; Emotions involved in tantrums
Feelings, labeling. *See* Labeling feelings
Fighting in front of children, 101–102
Firm voice
    creating structure and routine and, 137–138
    strategies for dealing with tantrums and, 164
Flexibility. *See also* Mental flexibility
    goodness of fit and, 93
    predictability and, 130–131
Fragile objects, touching, 57

Frequency of tantrums
    language delays and, 36–37
    red flags that may require professional assessment, 16, 17
Frustration
    avoiding emotions, 173
    emotional reactivity of parents and, 86–90
    modeling of, 146–147
    parent–child relationship and, 120
    settings for tantrums and, 201–204
    telling a child how to feel, 172–173

Game playing, 208
Gender, 4
Giving in, 165–166
Good cop/bad cop in parenting, 100–101. *See also* Parenting practices
Goodness of fit, 92–97
Gratitude expectations
    settings for tantrums and, 203–204
    strategies that don't work and, 177–178
Grief, 240

Habit creation, 196–197
Handling tantrums, 9. *See also* Responding to tantrums; Strategies for dealing with tantrums
Helping
    settings for tantrums and, 210
    strategies for dealing with tantrums and, 160–161
History of parents, 74–83
Hitting, 15
Holidays, 71
Home environment, 92–97. *See also* Family factors
Humor. *See also* Playfulness
    context of tantrums and, 42
    morning routines and, 185
    strategies for dealing with tantrums and, 158
Hunger
    mealtime routines and, 189–192
    as a possible cause, 33, 35

"I bet" phrase, 209–210
"I hate you" statements
    responding to, 88–90
    strategies that don't work and, 175–176
Ignoring behavior, 151–152
Illness, 216–218, 225–229
Imitation, 161
Impatience, 120
Impulse control, 15
Impulsivity. *See also* Characteristics that fuel tantrums
    example of, 60–61
    expectations and, 72

meeting children where they are, 63–66
overview, 49, 50–53
Inconsistency in parenting, 37–39. *See also*
    Limits; Parenting practices
Independence. *See also* Autonomy; Control
    desire for, 58–61
    distraction and, 160
Inhibitory control, 46–47, 50
Insecure attachment, 76. *See also* Attachment
Intelligence, 27
Intensity, 93. *See also* Temperament
Invalidation, 170–172. *See also* Validation of
    emotions
Irritation, 83–86

"**L** words." *See also* Limits; Love
    overview, 6, 105–111, 112
    predictability and, 129
    tricky situations and, 213
Labeling feelings. *See also* Emotions involved
    in tantrums
    leaving the house routines and, 188–189
    moving and, 219–220
    sickness and, 216–217
    strategies for dealing with tantrums and,
        155–156, 157
    strategies that don't work and, 178–179
Language development
    expressive language skills, 36–37, 47
    as a possible cause, 36–37
    receptive language skills, 36–37, 47
    self-injury and, 15–16
Language use by parents, 40–41
Learned behavior, 26–27
Leaving a setting, 211. *See also* Settings for
    tantrums
Leaving the house routines, 185–189
Limit testing. *See also* Limits; Power struggles
    explaining individual tantrums and, 25
    overview, 4
    personal histories of parents and, 78
    structure and, 131–132
Limits
    bedtime routines and, 196
    bending rules and, 134
    causes of tantrums and, 37–39
    connection and, 124
    extinction burst and, 133
    limit testing, 4, 25, 78, 131–132
    need for control and, 58–61
    overview, 6, 106, 112, 132–133
    personal histories of parents and, 78
    predictability and, 129
    safety and, 125–129
    separation of parents and, 223
    tricky situations and, 213
    validation of emotions and, 39–41
Listening, 163–166
Love
    overview, 6, 105–106, 112

predictability and, 129
tricky situations and, 213
Lying to children, 174

Management of tantrums, 9. *See also*
    Responding to tantrums; Strategies for
    dealing with tantrums
Manipulation, 26–27
Mealtime routines, 189–192. *See also* Eating
    patterns
Medication administration, 217–218. *See also*
    Illness
Meditations, 195. *See also* Mindfulness skills
Meetings, family, 136–137
Mental flexibility. *See also* Flexibility
    impulsivity and, 50
    rigidity and, 53–55
Mimicry, 145–147
Mindfulness skills
    bedtime routines and, 195
    emotional reactivity of parents and, 86–90
Mocking, 161
Modeling behavior
    mealtime routines and, 191
    settings for tantrums and, 203–204
    strategies for dealing with tantrums and,
        145–149
    strategies that don't work and, 174–175
Mommy and child special time
    new baby in the family and, 221–222
    reconnection and, 122
Mood, 93, 184. *See also* Temperament
Morning routines, 182–185
Moving, 218–220

Name calling, 178–179
Needs
    attachment and, 76
    context of tantrums and, 27
    of parents, 84–86
Negative consequences, 180–181
Negotiables, 131–132
Neural processing, 45. *See also* Brain
    development and processes
New places, 199. *See also* Settings for
    tantrums
Nonnegotiables, 131–132
Nonparental adults, tantrums with, 17
Nonverbal communication. *See also*
    Communication
    settings for tantrums and, 207
    strategies for dealing with tantrums and,
        157
Normalcy of tantrums. *See also*
    Developmental processes
    age for tantrums and, 4
    assumptions and, 8–9
    context of tantrums and, 17–22
    overview, 14–15, 20–22

Normalcy of tantrums (*continued*)
    reasons for tantrums and, 29–30
    strategies that don't work and, 180

Oversimplification, 25–29
Overstimulation, 199–200, 210–211

Parent–child relationship. *See also* Child;
        Connection; Parents
    foundation of, 113–116
    overview, 112
    reconnection and, 120–122
    repairing, 115–116
    repairing and reflecting after a tantrum
        and, 167–168
    safety and, 122–123
Parenting practices. *See also* Discipline;
        Parents
    appreciating mental efforts of child,
        48–49
    good cop/bad cop and, 100–101
    goodness of fit and, 92–97
    "L words" and, 105–111
    meeting children where they are, 63–66
    personal histories of parents and, 74–83
    as a possible cause, 37–40
    resources regarding, 231–240
    using fear, 109–111
Parents. *See also* Expectations; Family
        factors; Parent–child relationship;
        Parenting practices; Responding to
        tantrums
    emotional reactivity of, 86–90
    goodness of fit and, 92–97
    mealtime routines and, 191
    overview, 3, 67–70
    personal histories of, 74–83, 175
    pregnancy and, 220–221
    relationships between, 19, 100–102,
        223–224
    resources for, 231–236
    separation of, 223–224
    "Special Mommy/Daddy" time and, 122,
        221–222
    strategies that don't work and, 174–175
    stress levels and, 83–86
Parent's relationship with one another. *See
    also* Parents
    arguing in front of children and, 101–102
    context of tantrums and, 19
    good cop/bad cop and, 100–101
    separation and divorce, 223–224
Pausing before reacting, 9, 168–169. *See also*
        Responding to tantrums
Persistence, 93. *See also* Temperament
Personal histories of parents. *See* History of
        parents; Parents
Personality, 93, 96. *See also* Temperament

Perspective of the child, 142–144, 170–172
Perspective taking ability
    development of, 65–66
    empathy and, 63
Phases, 96–97
Phones, 151–152
Pictures, baby, 121
Places. *See* Settings for tantrums
Planning, 205. *See also* Preparation
Playfulness. *See also* Racing
    bath time routines and, 193
    leaving the house routines and, 189
    morning routines and, 185
    overview, 68–69
    settings for tantrums and, 208
    strategies for dealing with tantrums and,
        141
Police, threatening to call, 177
Poverty, 80–83
Power struggles. *See also* Limit testing
    mealtime routines and, 190, 191
    need for control and, 58–61
    responding to with playfulness, 68–69
    structure and, 129, 131–132
Precursors to tantrums, 32. *See also* Triggers
        for tantrums
Predictability
    expectations and, 71–72
    resiliency and, 130–131
    safety and, 125–129
    situations we can predict, 213–224
    situations we can't predict, 224–229
Predicting tantrums, 55
Pregnancy
    new baby in the family, 220–223
    by-the-way factors and, 103, 104–105
Preparation
    moving and, 218
    new baby in the family, 220
    settings for tantrums and, 206, 207
Preschool, 136
Preschool drop-offs
    parent–child relationship and, 118–120
    predictability and, 127–128
Presents, 203–204
Preventing tantrums. *See also* Strategies for
        dealing with tantrums
    "L words" and, 105–111
    ongoing, foundational strategies and,
        140–153
    prior to arriving, 204–207
    right before the tantrum, 153–162
    roles of parents in, 69–70
    tricky situations and, 213–224
Privilege. *See* Socioeconomic factors
Privileges, removal of, 180–181
Professional help
    red flags that may require professional
        assessment, 15–17
    resources regarding, 236

Props, 161
Punishment, 180–181. *See also* Discipline

Q-TIP acronym (Quit Taking It Personally)
  situations we can't predict and, 228
  strategies that don't work and, 175–176
Questions
  distraction and, 158–159
  settings for tantrums and, 208
Quit Taking It Personally (Q-TIP)
  situations we can't predict and, 228
  strategies that don't work and, 175–176

Racing. *See also* Playfulness
  distraction and, 159–160
  morning routines and, 185
  settings for tantrums and, 209
Rational explanations, 155
Reading together, 219
Reasoning with the child, 56–58
Reasons for tantrums. *See also* Context of the tantrum
  child's inability to state, 50–53
  goodness of fit and, 94–95
  overview, 5–6, 29–30
Receptive language skills, 36–37, 47. *See also* Language development
Red flags that may require professional assessment, 15–22
Reflecting feelings
  keeping it short, 156–157
  leaving the house routines and, 188–189
  settings for tantrums and, 210
  sickness and, 216–217
  strategies for dealing with tantrums and, 155–156
  after the tantrum, 167–168
Reflective functioning, 142–144
Regularity, 93. *See also* Temperament
Relationship between parents and toddlers or preschoolers. *See* Parent–child relationship
Relocation, 218–220
Repair, 167–168
Repetitive behaviors, 53–55
Resentment
  expectations and, 70–71
  mealtime routines and, 189–190
Resiliency
  predictability and, 130–131
  validation of emotions and, 39–41
Resources, 231–240
Responding to tantrums. *See also* Strategies for dealing with tantrums
  emotional reactivity and, 86–90
  "I hate you" statements and, 88–90
  influence of on the tantrum, 14–15
  "L words" and, 105–111

meeting children where they are, 63–66
  overview, 62, 67–70
  pausing before, 9, 168–169
  personal histories of parents and, 74–83
  playfulness and, 68–69
  strategies that don't work, 170–181
  stress levels and, 83–86
Response inhibition, 15
Responsibility
  mealtime routines and, 190–191
  settings for tantrums and, 210
Rewarding of tantrums, 37–39
Rewards
  morning routines and, 185
  settings for tantrums and, 206, 211
  using attention as, 149–151
Rigidity. *See also* Characteristics that fuel tantrums
  example of, 60–61
  meeting children where they are, 63–66
  overview, 49, 53–55
  predictability and, 130
Rituals
  moving and, 219
  overview, 53–55
  separation of parents and, 223–224
Routines
  bath time routines, 192–194
  bedtime routines, 180–181, 194–197
  bending rules and, 134
  consistent expectations and, 131–132
  creating, 134–138
  extinction burst and, 133
  leaving the house routines, 185–189
  mealtime routines, 189–192
  morning routines, 182–185
  moving and, 219–220
  overview, 53–55, 124
  personal histories of parents and, 78–79
  safety and, 125–129
  separation of parents and, 223–224
  travel and, 214–216
Rules. *See also* Expectations; Limits
  bending, 134
  creating, 135–136
  overview, 71, 132–133
  settings for tantrums and, 200–201, 202–203
Rushing, 187–189

Sadness, 27
Safety
  fear of parents and, 109
  parent–child relationship and, 122–123
  predictability and, 125–129
  strategies for dealing with tantrums and, 164–165
Sarcasm, 176–177

Schedules. *See also* Routines
  creating structure and routine and, 134–135
  expectations and, 71
  travel and, 214–216
School drop-offs
  parent–child relationship and, 118–120
  predictability and, 127–128
Secure attachment, 76, 116–120. *See also* Attachment
Self-awareness
  brain development and processes and, 47–48
  strategies for dealing with tantrums and, 141–142
Self-care of parents
  new baby in the family and, 223
  stress levels and, 84–86
Self-control. *See also* Emotional regulation
  brain development and processes and, 46–48
  impulsivity and, 50
  normalcy of tantrums and, 30
  overview, 28–29
  settings for tantrums and, 207, 211
Self-esteem, 92–93
Self-injury, 15–16
Self-soothing skills, 16
Sensory inputs, 200
Sensory threshold, 93. *See also* Temperament
Separation of parents, 223–224
Settings for tantrums
  after leaving, 211
  overview, 198–204
  prior to arriving, 204–207
  rules and, 200–201
  while at the setting, 207–211
Severity of tantrums, 36–37
Sex differences, 4
Shame, 202–203
Shopping, 199–200, 205–206
Siblings
  expectations and, 71
  new baby in the family, 220–223
  role of, 97–98
Sickness, 216–218, 225–229
Silliness, 141
Sleep patterns. *See also* Bedtime routines
  morning routines and, 183
  as a possible cause, 33, 35
  resources regarding, 234–235
  sickness and, 217
Sleepiness, 33, 35
Smart phones, 151–152
Snacking, 192. *See also* Eating patterns; Mealtime routines
Social factors
  comparisons, 71
  goodness of fit and, 93–95
  norms, 71
  personal histories of parents and, 82

Socioeconomic factors, 80–83
Songs
  leaving the house routines and, 188
  morning routines and, 185
  settings for tantrums and, 209
"Special Mommy/Daddy" time
  new baby in the family and, 221–222
  reconnection and, 122
Special occasions, 71
Spoiling children, 80–81
Stimulation, 199–200
Strategic attention
  giving children credit, 154
  leaving the house routines and, 189
  morning routines and, 185
  settings for tantrums and, 208–209
  strategies for dealing with tantrums and, 149–153
Strategies for dealing with tantrums. *See also* Handling tantrums; Management of tantrums; Preventing tantrums; Responding to tantrums
  being present and listening, 163–166
  child factors, 142–145
  choices and, 161–162
  distraction, 158–161
  emotionality and, 154–158
  giving children credit, 153–154
  modeling and, 145–149
  ongoing, foundational strategies, 140–153
  overview, 6–7, 139–140
  parent factors, 140–142
  pausing before reacting, 168–169
  predictability and, 129
  right before the tantrum, 153–162
  strategies that don't work, 170–181
  during the tantrum, 162–166
  after the tantrum, 167–168
  using attention, 149–153
Stress levels
  responding to tantrums and, 83–86
  settings for tantrums and, 201–204, 207
  situations we can't predict, 224–229
  tricky situations and, 213–214
Structure
  bedtime routines and, 195–196
  bending rules and, 134
  consistent expectations and, 131–132
  creating, 134–138
  extinction burst and, 133
  "L words" and, 106
  morning routines and, 183–184
  moving and, 219–220
  overview, 124
  personal histories of parents and, 78–79
  safety and, 125–129
  setting limits and, 132–133
  settings for tantrums and, 206
Successes, recognizing, 154
Surprises, 130–131
Sweets, 191. *See also* Eating patterns

Tantrum interactions. *See also* Responding
    to tantrums
    family factors and, 97–102
    overview, 67–68
    personal histories of parents and, 74–83
    by-the-way factors and, 102–105
Tantrums. *See also* Causes of tantrums
    assumptions regarding, 8–9
    extinction burst and, 133
    oversimplification of, 25–29
    overview, 5, 22, 24–29
    reasons for the occurance of, 5–6
    red flags that may require professional
        assessment, 15–17
Technology, 205–206
Temperament
    goodness of fit and, 92–97
    overview, 93
    settings for tantrums and, 199
Temptations, 199–200
Theory of mind, 65–66
Thinking ahead, 143–144
Thinking brain, 45–46. *See also* Brain
    development and processes
Threats, 177
Throwing, 15
Time with child, special
    new baby in the family and, 221–222
    reconnection and, 122
Time-outs, 106–109, 180–181
Timing tantrums
    egocentrism, 61–63
    red flags that may require professional
        assessment, 16
Tiredness, 33, 35
Tone of voice. *See also* Firm voice; Yelling
    creating structure and routine and,
        137–138
    settings for tantrums and, 210
    strategies for dealing with tantrums and,
        164
Touch, 164–165
Touching fragile objects, 57
Transitions
    bath time routines and, 193
    leaving the house routines and, 187–189
    new baby in the family and, 220–223
    as a possible cause, 35–36
    separation of parents and, 223–224
Traumatic events, 224–229, 232
Travel, 71, 214–216
Treats, 203–204
Tricky situations. *See also* Events
    moving, 218–220
    new baby in the family, 220–223
    overview, 212–213
    resources regarding, 240
    separation of parents, 223–224
    sickness, 216–218
    that we can predict, 213–224

that we can't predict, 224–229
travel, 214–216
Triggers for tantrums. *See also* Antecedents;
    Causes of tantrums; Context of the
    tantrum
    "ABCs" of tantrums, 17–22
    behavioral chain analysis and, 32–33, 34*f*
    multiple factors and, 32–33, 34*f*
    overview, 23–24, 31–33, 42
    by-the-way factors and, 102–105
Trust
    fear of parents and, 109
    predictability and, 127
Two-parent families, 98–102. *See also* Family
    factors

Understanding
    safety and, 123
    secure attachment and, 117–120
    settings for tantrums and, 207, 210–211
    strategies for dealing with tantrums and,
        155–156
Unfamiliar places, 199–200. *See also* Settings
    for tantrums

Vacations, 71, 214–216
Validation of emotions
    causes of tantrums and, 39–41
    moving and, 219–220
    strategies that don't work and, 170–172
Verbal communication. *See also*
    Communication
    settings for tantrums and, 207
    strategies for dealing with tantrums and,
        157
Visual aids
    leaving the house routines and, 188
    morning routines and, 184–185
Visualization, 121–122
Voice, tone of. *See* Tone of voice

Warning signs
    context of tantrums and, 17–22
    red flags that may require professional
        assessment, 15–17
Warnings to the child, 188
Wealth, 80–83
Weekends, 71
Working memory, 46–47
Writing exercises, 121–122

Yelling
    age for tantrums and, 4
    creating structure and routine and,
        137–138
    emotional reactivity of parents and, 87–88

About the Author

Rebecca Schrag Hershberg, PhD, is a clinical psychologist and founder of Little House Calls Psychological Services, which specializes in helping kids and parents confronting a range of common early childhood challenges. Dr. Hershberg has held leadership positions at a national nonprofit organization serving children and a hospital-based infant and toddler preventive mental health program. She has taught in the Department of Pediatrics at the Albert Einstein College of Medicine and has presented numerous seminars and workshops for parents. She lives in the New York City area with her husband and two young sons.